Fast Facts for Healthcare
Professionals

Epilepsy in Adults

Phil Tittensor RNLD DipN NIP MSc
Chairperson, Epilepsy Nurses Association (ESNA)
Consultant Nurse for the Epilepsies
The Royal Wolverhampton NHS Trust
Honorary Lecturer, University of Wolverhampton
Wolverhampton, UK

Sheila Shepley RGN BSc PhD
Advanced Nurse Practitioner Clinician
Walton Centre NHS Foundation Trust
Betsi Cadwalader University Health Board BCUHB
Liverpool, UK

Martin J Brodie MB ChB MRCP MD FRCP
Chief Medical Officer and Immediate Past President
International Bureau for Epilepsy (IBE)
Professor of Medicine and Clinical Pharmacology
Epilepsy Unit, University of Glasgow
Glasgow, UK

Declaration of Independence
This book is as balanced and practical as we can make it.
Ideas for improvement are always welcome: fastfacts@karger.com

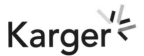

HEALTHCARE

Fast Facts: Epilepsy in Adults
First published 2023

Text © 2023 Phil Tittensor, Sheila Shepley, Martin J Brodie
© 2023 in this edition S. Karger Publishers Ltd

S. Karger Publishers Ltd, Elizabeth House, Queen Street, Abingdon,
Oxford OX14 3LN, UK
Tel: +44 (0)1235 523233

Book orders can be placed by telephone or email, or via the website.
Please telephone +41 61 306 1440 or email orders@karger.com
To order via the website, please go to karger.com

Fast Facts is a trademark of S. Karger Publishers Ltd.

A CIP record for this title is available from the British Library.

ISBN 978-3-318-07081-1

Tittensor P (Phil)
Fast Facts: Epilepsy in Adults/
Phil Tittensor, Sheila Shepley, Martin J Brodie

Typesetting by Amnet, Chennai, India.
Printed in the UK with Xpedient Print.

List of abbreviations

ACT: acceptance commitment therapy

AMPA: α-amino-3-hydroxy-5-methyl-4-isoxazolepropionic acid

ASM: antiseizure medication

AV: atrioventricular

BMD: bone mineral density

BRV: brivaracetam

CBT: cognitive behavioral therapy

CBZ: carbamazepine

CEN: cenobamate

CI: confidence interval

CLB: clobazam

CNS: central nervous system

CT: computed tomography

CYP450: cytochrome P450

DBS: deep-brain stimulation

DEXA: dual-energy X-ray absorptiometry

DRESS: drug reaction with eosinophilia and systemic symptoms

DRN: dorsal raphe nuclei

DS: Dravet syndrome

ECG: electrocardiogram

EEG: electroencephalography/electroencephalogram

ESL: eslicarbazepine acetate

ESM: ethosuximide

FBM: felbamate

GABA: gamma-aminobutyric acid

GBP: gabapentin

GGE: genetic generalized epilepsies

GTCS: generalized tonic–clonic seizure(s)

HIV: human immunodeficiency virus

HRT: hormone replacement therapy

ID: intellectual disability

IGE: idiopathic generalized epilepsy

ILAE: International League Against Epilepsy

IUD: intrauterine device

LC: locus coeruleus

LCM: lacosamide

LEV: levetiracetam

LGS: Lennox–Gastaut syndrome

LTG: lamotrigine

MCM: major congenital malformation

MRI: magnetic resonance imaging

MRS: magnetic resonance spectroscopy

NCSE: non-convulsive status epilepticus

NMDA: N-methyl-D-aspartate

NTS: nucleus tractus solitarius

OCP: oral contraceptive pill

OXC: oxcarbazepine

PB: phenobarbital

PBN: parabrachial nucleus

PER: perampanel

PET: positron emission tomography

PGB: pregabalin

PHT: phenytoin

PNES: psychogenic non-epileptic seizures

PPI: patient and public involvement

PRM: primidone

PSP: priority setting partnership

RFN: rufinamide

RNS: responsive neural stimulation

SE: status epilepticus

SmPC: summary of product characteristics

SPECT: single photon emission computed tomography

STP: stiripentol

SUDEP: sudden unexpected death in epilepsy

SV2A: synaptic vesicle glycoprotein 2A

TGB: tigabine

TPM: topiramate

TSC: tuberous sclerosis complex

VGB: vigabatrin

VNS: vagus nerve stimulation

VPA: sodium valproate

ZNS: zonisamide

Introduction

Epilepsy is the most common serious neurological condition in the world. However, as it is not a homogeneous disease, it is preferable to use the term 'epilepsies', as this better describes a grouping of conditions that share a propensity for an individual to experience sudden unprovoked seizures because of abnormal electrical activity within the brain. While some epilepsies spontaneously remit, some are lifelong and others have a variable prognosis. Complicating the picture are seizures that superficially look like epilepsy but have a psychological cause (psychogenic non-epileptic seizures).

Seizures can affect people of all ages and ethnic backgrounds. They can be dangerous, with sudden unexpected death in epilepsy (SUDEP) occurring in 1 in 1000 people with epilepsy; perhaps as many as 1 in 100 with medically intractable seizures. Psychiatric and other comorbidities are common, and seizures are much more likely to occur in people with intellectual disability, where there can be a complex interplay between epilepsy, treatment and behavior.

With a growing array of targeted therapies, specific syndromes need to be identified and characterized so that these treatments can be offered to individuals who may derive benefit from them. Despite this, the proportion of people with seizures resistant to antiseizure medication (ASM) remains stubbornly static at around 30%. It is yet to be seen whether the latest ASM can have a significant effect on this figure. Surgical options exist for some people, and there have been significant advances in neurostimulation techniques over the last few years, including novel devices and new algorithms for vagus nerve stimulation.

In this resource, we focus on the management of epilepsy in adults. Its sister publication *Fast Facts: Epilepsy in Children and Adolescents* is also available, together with an online learning program. We hope to have produced a book that is accessible for both healthcare professionals and people with epilepsy. The aim is to provide a succinct and practical resource that will help clinicians investigate, diagnose and treat adults with a wide variety of seizure disorders and also to help people with epilepsy better understand and manage their condition.

1 Epidemiology and prognosis

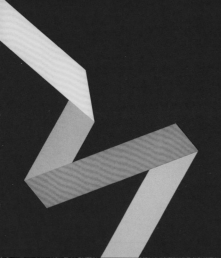

HEALTHCARE

Incidence and prevalence

Epilepsy is the most common serious neurological condition. It affects nearly 50 million people of all ages worldwide.[1] The pooled results of a systematic review and meta-analysis in 2020 showed the overall incidence of epilepsy worldwide to be 61.4 per 100000 person-years. The incidence was higher in low- and middle-income countries than in high-income countries (139 versus 48.9 per 100000 person-years, respectively), with greater exposure to perinatal risk factors and higher rates of CNS infections and traumatic brain injury thought to explain the differences.[2]

A correlation exists between the prevalence of epilepsy and certain measures of socioeconomic deprivation, notably income, employment, and health deprivation and disability. For example, the population prevalence of epilepsy in England ranges from around 4.3 per 1000 in certain counties of the wealthier south-east to 11.6 per 1000 in the socioeconomically deprived north-west town of Blackpool.[3] In the USA, studies show racial and economic disparities exist in epilepsy diagnosis, treatment and overall care.[4] Differences in access to healthcare are likely to be one explanation for these disparities.

Incidence varies greatly with age, with high rates in early childhood, low levels in early adult life and a second peak in people aged over 65 years (Figure 1.1).[5] In recent years, there has been a fall in the number of children affected as well as a sharp rise in epilepsy in the elderly. Indeed, old age has now become the most common time in life to develop the condition.

Prognosis

The epilepsies are a heterogeneous group of conditions. Prognosis depends on the underlying cause and syndromic diagnosis, but most people will have a good prognosis. In many people – particularly children – the condition will remit, although a substantial proportion will have epilepsy all their lives.

Overall, 60–70% of people with epilepsy become seizure free after treatment with antiseizure medication (ASM),[6] and some individuals can remain in remission after subsequent drug withdrawal, implying that the epileptogenic causes have truly remitted. The other 30–40%

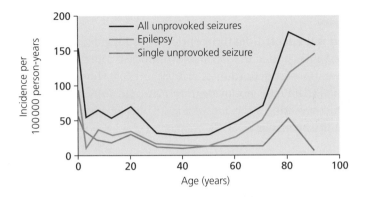

Figure 1.1 Incidence of single unprovoked seizures, epilepsy and all unprovoked seizures in Iceland between December 1995 and February 1999. Age-specific incidence of all unprovoked seizures was highest in the first year of life (130 per 100 000 person-years) and in those over 65 years old (110.5 per 100 000 person-years). Reproduced from Olafsson et al. 2005, with permission from Elsevier.[5]

continue to have seizures with varying degrees of frequency and severity.

Some people become – and remain – seizure free on initiation of the first ASM, while in others the disorder may follow a more 'remitting–relapsing' course, fluctuating between periods of seizure freedom and recurrence. A good example of this is temporal lobe epilepsy due to mesial temporal sclerosis, where patients often achieve seizure freedom following initiation of ASM, but relapse months to years later, with a poor response to additional medication.[7]

Factors that indicate a poor prognosis for seizure control include:

- poor response to the initial ASM
- symptomatic causes
- high seizure frequency before ASM
- generalized tonic–clonic seizures (GTCS)
- generalized epileptiform activity on the electroencephalogram (EEG)
- family history of epilepsy
- comorbid psychiatric history.

Mortality

Sudden unexpected death in epilepsy. As long ago as 1854, Delasiauve recognized that people with epilepsy could die suddenly. However, the first definition of sudden unexpected death in epilepsy (SUDEP) was not made until 1997. This was further refined in 2011, incorporating a classification system to establish the likelihood of a fatality being due to SUDEP (Table 1.1).[8] A large Swedish

TABLE 1.1

Unified SUDEP definition and classification

Definite SUDEP
Sudden, unexpected, witnessed or unwitnessed, non-traumatic and non-drowning death, occurring in benign circumstances in an individual with epilepsy, with or without evidence for a seizure and excluding documented status epilepticus (seizure duration ≥30 minutes or seizures without recovery in between). Postmortem examination does not reveal a cause of death.

Definite SUDEP Plus
Satisfying the definition of definite SUDEP if a concomitant condition other than epilepsy is identified before or after death, if the death may have been due to the combined effect of both conditions, and if postmortem examination or direct observations/recordings of terminal event did not prove the concomitant condition to be the cause of death.

Probable SUDEP/Probable SUDEP Plus
Same as definite SUDEP but without postmortem evidence. The victim should have died unexpectedly while in a reasonable state of health, during normal activities and in benign circumstances without a known structural cause of death.

Possible SUDEP
A competing cause of death is present.

Near-SUDEP/Near-SUDEP Plus
A patient with epilepsy survives resuscitation for more than 1 hour after a cardiorespiratory arrest that has no structural cause identified after investigation.

Not SUDEP
A clear cause of death is known.

Unclassified
Incomplete information available; not possible to classify.

population-based study used these criteria to establish that the incidence of definite/probable SUDEP was 1.2 per 1000 person-years.[9]

Table 1.2 shows the main risk factors for SUDEP. GTCS, with or without focal onset, is the biggest single risk factor. The presence of multiple risks increases mortality exponentially. For example, having at least one GTCS in the previous year and not sharing a bedroom with someone confers a 67-fold increased risk of SUDEP compared with not having a GTCS and sharing a bedroom.[10] Less relevant risks include generalized epilepsies (no significant difference compared with focal epilepsies when GTCS are removed), educational level and mental health disorders.

Women with epilepsy who are pregnant (or have recently given birth) are also vulnerable to SUDEP, with the UK's MBRRACE national enquiry flagging a doubling of SUDEP deaths among this group in 2016–2018.[11]

Other causes of death in people with epilepsy. People with epilepsy have a much higher risk of accidents, drowning, burns, aspiration, pneumonia, status epilepticus (SE) and suicide than the general population. Many risk factors associated with epilepsy mortality are known to be modifiable,[12] and communicating these risks to people with epilepsy has been shown to help with risk reduction.[13,14] Previous research suggested 42% of epilepsy deaths could be potentially

TABLE 1.2

Risk factors for SUDEP

Risk factor	Increased risk compared with controls
Nocturnal GTCS in last year	15-fold
GTCS	10-fold
Nocturnal GTCS	9-fold
Living alone	5-fold
Sharing a household but sleeping alone	2-fold
Substance abuse/alcohol dependence	2-fold

Adapted from Sveinsson et al. 2020.[10]

avoidable[15] while more recent studies suggest this figure could be significantly higher (up to 80% preventable).[16] Not taking steps to address epilepsy mortality risks can lead to premature deaths in people who are often young and otherwise healthy.

It is particularly noteworthy that in the UK between 2018 and 2020, the Learning Disabilities Mortality Review (LeDeR) Programme reported epilepsy as one of the most frequently recorded avoidable medical causes of deaths among adults with intellectual disability (ID).[17]

Socioeconomic costs

Epilepsy carries a significant socioeconomic burden. In a large cohort study in Denmark, 10000 of 40000 people with diagnosed epilepsy were compared with 23000 controls.[18] People with epilepsy tended to have a lower level of education, be less likely to be married (and have a higher incidence of divorce) and consequently be more likely to live alone. This is significant when considering the risk factors discussed above. In addition, people with epilepsy were more likely to be unemployed, receive disability benefits and, even if in employment, have a lower income than controls.

Epilepsy also confers a significant cost to healthcare systems. A European study published in 2014 estimated that the direct mean annual epilepsy-related costs of a patient with drug-resistant epilepsy was €4485, compared with €1926 for patients with drug-responsive epilepsy.[19] The additional costs were divided between ASM, additional tests and, most significantly, increased hospitalization. The overall direct cost of focal epilepsy in adults was estimated at €3850 per patient per year.

Key points – epidemiology and prognosis

- A systematic review and meta-analysis found an overall global incidence of epilepsy of 61.4 per 100 000 person-years, with higher incidence in low- and middle-income countries.
- The incidence of epilepsy peaks in early childhood and again in people aged over 65 years; older age is now the most common time of life to develop the condition.
- Most people with epilepsy will have a good prognosis.
- GTCS, with or without focal onset, is the biggest single risk factor for SUDEP.
- The socioeconomic cost of epilepsy is significant, affecting both individuals with epilepsy and healthcare systems.

References

1. World Health Organization. Epilepsy. A Public health Imperative. World Health Organization, 2019. www. who.int/publications/i/item/ epilepsy-a-public-health-imperative, last accessed 20 April 2022.

2. Beghi E. The epidemiology of epilepsy. *Neuroepidemiology* 2020;54:185–91.

3. Steer S, Pickrell, WO, Kerr MP, Thomas RH. Epilepsy prevalence and socioeconomic deprivation in England. *Epilepsia* 2014;55:1634–41.

4. Blank LJ. Socioeconomic disparities in epilepsy care. *Curr Opin Neurol* 2022;35: 169–74.

5. Olafsson E, Ludvigsson P, Hesdorffer D et al. Incidence of unprovoked seizures and epilepsy in Iceland and assessment of the epilepsy syndrome classification: a prospective study. *Lancet Neurol* 2005;4:627–34.

6. Kwan P, Brodie MJ. Early identification of refractory epilepsy. *N Engl J Med* 2000; 342:314–19.

7. Berg AT. The natural history of mesial temporal lobe epilepsy. *Curr Opin Neurol* 2008;21:173–8.

8. Nashef L, So EL, Ryvlin P et al. Unifying the definitions of sudden unexpected death in epilepsy. *Epilepsia* 2012;53:227–33.

9. Sveinsson O, Andersson T, Carlasson S, Tomson T. The incidence of SUDEP. A nationwide population-based cohort study. *Neurology* 2017;89:170–7.

10. Sveinsson O, Andersson T, Mattsson P et al. Clinical risk factors in SUDEP. A nationwide population-based case-control study. *Neurology* 2020;94: e419–29.

11. Knight M, Bunch K, Tuffnell D et al., on behalf of MBRRACE-UK. *Saving Lives, Improving Mothers' Care. Lessons learned to inform maternity care from the UK and Ireland Confidential Enquiries into Maternal Deaths and Morbidity 2016–18.* Healthcare Quality Improvement Partnership and National Perinatal Epidemiology Unit, University of Oxford, 2020. www.npeu. ox.ac.uk/assets/downloads/ mbrrace-uk/reports/maternal-report-2020/MBRRACE-UK_ Maternal_Report_Dec_2020_ v10_ONLINE_VERSION_1404. pdf, last accessed 20 April 2022.

12. McCabe J, McLean B, Henley W et al. Sudden unexpected death in epilepsy (SUDEP) and seizure safety: modifiable and non-modifiable risk factors differences between primary and secondary care. *Epilepsy Behav* 2021;115:107637.

13. Smart C, Page G, Shankar R, Newman C. Keep safe: the when, why and how of epilepsy risk communication. *Seizure* 2020;78:136–49.

14. Shankar R, Henley W, Boland C et al. Decreasing the risk of sudden unexpected death in epilepsy: structured communication of risk factors for premature mortality in people with epilepsy. *Eur J Neurol* 2018;25:1121–7.

15. Hanna NJ, Black M, Sander JW et al. National Sentinel Clinical Audit of Epilepsy-Related Death. Report 2002. Epilepsy Bereaved, 2002. www. sudep.org/sites/default/files/ nationalsentinelreport1.pdf, last accessed 20 April 2022.

16. Mbizvo GK Schnier C, Simpson CR, Chin RFM. A national study of epilepsy-related deaths in Scotland: trends, mechanisms, and avoidable deaths. *Epilepsia* 2021;62:2667–84.

17. University of Bristol. *The Learning Disabilities Mortality Review (LeDeR) Programme. Annual Report 2020.* University of Bristol, 2021. www.england.nhs.uk/ wp-content/uploads/2021/06/ LeDeR-bristol-annual-report-2020.pdf, last accessed 20 April 2022.

18. Jennum P, Christensen J, Ibsen R, Kjellberg J. Long-term socioeconomic consequences and health care costs of childhood and adolescent-onset epilepsy. *Epilepsia* 2016;57:1078–85.

19. de Zélicourt M, de Toffol B, Vespignani H et al. Management of focal epilepsy in adults treated with polytherapy in France: the direct cost of drug resistance (ESPERA study). *Seizure* 2014;23:349–56.

2 Classification and causes of seizures, epilepsy types and syndromes

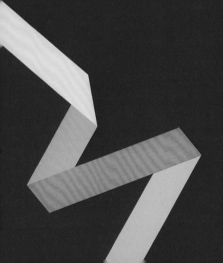

The 2017 International League Against Epilepsy (ILAE) revised Classification of the Epilepsies includes a three-level seizure classification framework (Figure 2.1) to aid diagnosis.[1-5] The first level identifies seizure types (focal, generalized and unknown onset), the second level considers epilepsy types (focal, generalized, combined focal and generalized, and unknown) and the third level considers specific epilepsy syndromes. However, it must be remembered that it is not possible to arrive at a syndromic diagnosis for all people with epilepsy. The etiologies sit alongside the three levels and encompass structural, genetic, infectious, metabolic, immune and unknown categories. Some epilepsies can be attributed to more than one etiology. Overlapping this framework are comorbidities (learning, psychological, behavioral, etc.) associated with seizures and epilepsy (see Chapter 9).

Seizure types

A seizure is a symptom and represents the clinical manifestation of an abnormal and excessive synchronized discharge of a set of cortical neurons in the brain. Establishing the type(s) of seizure has important implications for:
- choice of investigations
- selection of ASM
- likelihood of an underlying cerebral lesion
- prognosis
- possible genetic transmission.

Depending on the pattern of neuron involvement, the clinical features of a seizure consist of a wide range of sudden and transitory abnormal phenomena, which may include alterations of consciousness, or motor, sensory, autonomic or cognitive events (see Figure 2.1). Minor seizures are often more important than major bilateral tonic–clonic seizures for determining an appropriate diagnosis, and for diagnostic tests and management strategies.

Figure 2.1 ILAE classification of the epilepsies. Adapted from Scheffer et al. 2017[1] and Fisher et al. 2017.[2]

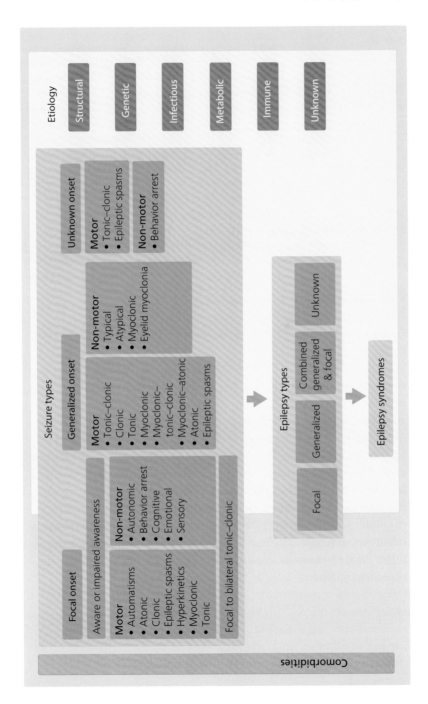

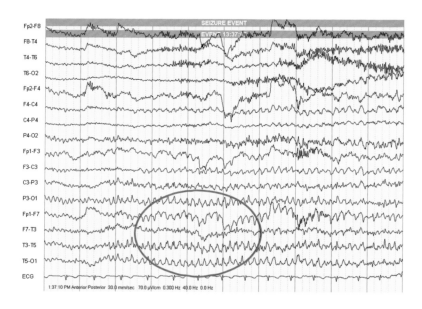

Figure 2.2 EEG showing a focal seizure over the left temporal area (circled).

Focal seizures (previously called partial seizures) originate from one hemisphere within the brain – the frontal, temporal (Figure 2.2), parietal or occipital lobes. Seizures can be subdivided into those where awareness is retained (focal aware seizures) and those where it is not (focal impaired-awareness seizures). This differentiation is essential for identifying individuals whose safety may be compromised by loss of awareness during their seizures. Focal seizures can also be classified according to their clinical manifestations, such as focal motor and non-motor onset, and can spread rapidly to other cortical areas through neuronal networks, resulting in focal to bilateral tonic–clonic seizures (Figure 2.3). The first symptom of a focal seizure, sometimes called an aura, is vitally important for localizing and lateralizing the epileptogenic focus.

Focal aware seizures. The signs and symptoms of focal aware seizures depend on the site of origin of the abnormal electrical discharges. For example, those arising from the motor cortex can cause epileptic spasms and hyperkinetic (agitated thrashing or leg pedaling movements) or unilateral clonic movements.

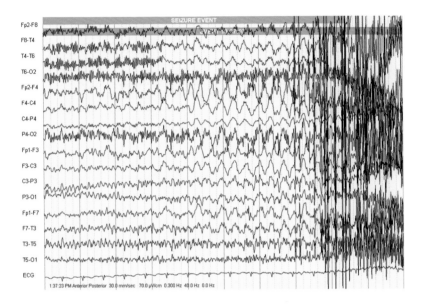

Figure 2.3 EEG showing a bilateral tonic–clonic seizure following from the focal-onset seizure in Figure 2.2.

Seizures arising from non-motor regions may produce autonomic, emotional, sensory, cognitive or behavioral symptoms. It is important to encourage more detailed free text descriptors (Table 2.1) from the person with epilepsy to help to identify motor and non-motor signs and symptoms before and after seizures.

Focal impaired-awareness seizures are the most common seizure type in adults with epilepsy. Focal impaired-awareness seizures originating from the temporal lobe may start with a focal aware seizure (some people consider this a useful warning), which rapidly progresses to a complete loss or reduction of awareness. Seizures typically last 1–4 minutes. During that time, the person may appear awake, but lose contact with their environment; they do not respond normally to instructions or questions. They usually stare and either remain motionless or exhibit impaired function, engaging in repetitive semi-purposeful behavior called automatisms, including facial grimacing, gesturing, chewing, lip smacking, snapping fingers, repeating words or phrases, walking, running or even undressing. The person cannot remember behaving in this manner. If restrained, they

23

TABLE 2.1

Common descriptors of behaviors during and after seizures

Type of behavior	Common descriptors
Cognitive	Acalculia, aphasia, attention impairment, déjà vu or jamais vu, dissociation, dysphasia, forced thinking, hallucinations, illusions, impaired memory, impaired responsiveness
Automatisms	Aggression, eye-blinking, head-nodding, manual, oral-facial, pedaling, pelvic thrusting, perseveration, running (cursive), sexual, undressing, vocalization/speech, walking
Emotional or affective	Agitation, anger, anxiety, crying (dacrystic), fear, laughing (gelastic), paranoia, pleasure
Autonomic	Asystole, bradycardia, erection, flushing, gastrointestinal, hyper/hypoventilation, nausea/vomiting, pallor, palpitations, piloerection, respiratory changes, tachycardia
Motor	Dysarthria, dystonic, fencer's posture (figure of 4), incoordination, Jacksonian, paralysis, paresis, versive
Sensory	Auditory, gustatory, hot-cold sensations, olfactory, somatosensory, vestibular, visual
Laterality	Left, right, bilateral

may become hostile or aggressive. After the seizure they are often sleepy and confused and complain of a headache. This postictal state can last from minutes to hours.

Focal impaired-awareness seizures originating from the frontal lobe are the second most common type of seizures seen at epilepsy centers during presurgical evaluation for drug-resistant epilepsy. Because of the large size of the frontal lobe (40% of the entire cerebral cortex), a variety of clinical manifestations is seen in seizures arising from the different subregions. In general, frontal lobe seizures are shorter in duration than seizures arising from the temporal lobe, with a preponderance to cluster during nighttime. They have a strong motor component and consciousness is often preserved. Through involvement of the motor areas, there may be unilateral clonic movements of the extremities, trunk or face. Asymmetric tonic seizures are seen, classically with tonic arm extension and elevation, and forced head deviation to the side of the extended arm, referred to as a 'fencer's posture'.

In other forms, the seizures are described as 'hyperkinetic', with sudden and sometimes explosive onset of complex and violent behavioral automatisms. The person may jump around, rotate or pound on objects, and commonly exhibit cycling or stepping movements. Motor features are often accompanied by vocalization, mainly in the form of a scream or grunts, though this vocalization can be part of understandable speech. As frontal lobe seizures often appear bizarre, they are frequently misdiagnosed as psychogenic non-epileptic seizures (PNES) (see Chapter 10).

Focal to generalized bilateral tonic–clonic seizures. Both focal aware and focal impaired-awareness seizures can lead to bilateral tonic–clonic seizures (previously called secondary GTCS), although the aura is often not recognized by the person afterwards. It quickly leads to bilateral tonic–clonic movements, sometimes with lateral tongue or mouth biting and/or urinary incontinence. The typical duration is 2–3 minutes, with jerking movements slowing, becoming more asynchronous and larger in amplitude as the seizure progresses. When the jerking stops, the person will become deeply unresponsive for a short while, usually making strenuous breathing noises. Cyanosis may occur. The person may exhibit postictal focal impaired-awareness activity and appear confused. Keeping this sequence of events in mind is very important when differentiating between focal-onset seizures and primary GTCS as well as PNES.

Generalized-onset seizures are characterized by widespread involvement of bilateral cortical regions at the outset and are usually accompanied by impaired consciousness. The familiar tonic–clonic seizure (previously called 'grand mal') often starts with a cry. The patient suddenly falls to the ground and exhibits typical bilateral tonic–clonic movements, sometimes with lateral tongue or mouth biting and/or urinary incontinence. The absence of an aura delineates these from focal-onset bilateral tonic–clonic seizures, though they may be preceded by a series of myoclonic jerks or absences in some generalized epilepsy syndromes.

Other types of generalized-onset motor seizures include tonic, clonic, myoclonic, myoclonic–tonic–clonic, myoclonic–atonic, atonic and epileptic spasms. Generalized-onset non-motor seizures include typical and atypical absence seizures and eyelid myoclonia.

Absence seizures (previously called 'petit mal') usually start in childhood. At least 40% remit during adolescence.

Typical absence seizures usually last 5–10 seconds. They manifest as sudden onset of staring and impaired consciousness, with or without eye blinking and lip smacking. The EEG typically shows a 3-Hz spike-and-wave pattern (Figure 2.4). There is a strong genetic component.

Atypical absence seizures usually begin before 5 years of age in conjunction with other generalized seizure types and learning disability. They last longer than typical absence seizures and are often associated with changes in muscle tone.

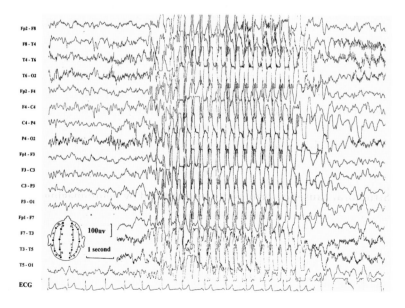

Figure 2.4 EEG showing the 3-Hz spike-and-wave pattern of a typical absence seizure, with characteristic abrupt onset and cessation.

Myoclonic seizures consist of sudden brief muscle contractions, either singly or in clusters, that can affect any muscle group.

Clonic seizures are characterized by rhythmic or semi-rhythmic muscle contractions, typically involving the upper extremities, neck and face.

Tonic seizures cause sudden stiffening of the extensor muscles, often associated with impaired consciousness and falling to the ground.

Atonic seizures (also called drop attacks) produce sudden loss of muscle tone with instantaneous collapse (imagine a marionette puppet having its strings cut), often resulting in facial or other injuries.

Epilepsy syndromes

Epilepsy syndromes are defined by groups of characteristic clinical features related to age at seizure onset, family history of epilepsy, seizure type(s) and neurological signs and symptoms, aided by appropriate investigations, including EEG and brain imaging (see Chapter 3).

Epilepsy syndromes can be focal or generalized in nature, with generalized epilepsy syndromes classified as genetic generalized epilepsies (GGE), though the older name idiopathic generalized epilepsy (IGE) is still regularly used and recognized as a useful term by the ILAE.

Diagnosing an epileptic syndrome enables clinicians to define the likely prognosis, provide reasonable genetic counseling and choose the most appropriate ASM. Most epilepsy syndromes start in childhood and continue into adulthood (see *Fast Facts: Epilepsy in Children and Adolescents*) (Table 2.2).

Etiologies

Structural causes of seizures can be identified by neuroimaging of the brain. Signs and symptoms before a seizure may give the clinician an indication of where the anatomic abnormality is located (see Chapter 3). Structural abnormality may be acquired: for example, a previous head injury, stroke, birth injury, tumor or brain infection. Equally, a person with epilepsy may have been born with an anatomic defect with a genetic cause. Some epilepsy types can be attributed to more than one cause: for example, tuberous sclerosis and neurofibromatosis are genetic conditions that usually grow

TABLE 2.2

Epilepsy syndromes originating in adolescents and adults

- GGE/IGE
- Juvenile absence epilepsy
- Juvenile myoclonic epilepsy
- Epilepsy with GTCS alone
- Autosomal dominant epilepsy with auditory features
- Other familial temporal lobe epilepsies (such as mesial temporal lobe including hippocampus)

Adapted from epilepsydiagnosis.org.

benign tumors (structural) in the brain that may provoke seizures. The structural cause takes precedence.

Acute and/or chronic infection within the CNS can result in brain damage and seizures (most common in developing countries). Infectious causes include HIV, tuberculosis, malaria, bacterial meningitis and viral meningitis. More widespread damage to brain structure is more likely to cause difficult-to-control seizures. Treating the infection quickly is the most important therapeutic strategy.

Immune conditions can result in seizures when the body responds to infection by producing antibodies against its own tissues (antibody-mediated etiology). Immune causes are diagnosed when there is evidence of autoimmune-mediated CNS inflammation in the brain leading to epilepsy (for example, Rasmussen syndrome). The priority for clinicians is to treat the cause of autoimmune-mediated seizures and epilepsy.

Genetic etiologies may be attributed to either chromosomal or molecular abnormalities. Some chromosomal abnormalities are recognized by the seizure type and EEG features.

Well-replicated molecular genetic studies derived from appropriately designed family studies have become the basis of diagnostic testing. Table 2.3 lists some of the genes associated with epilepsy syndromes.

Many genetic factors can lead to epilepsy, including:

- inherited gene abnormalities – autosomal dominant, autosomal recessive and Mendelian inheritance
- acquired gene abnormalities – de novo, sporadic, mosaicism, germline and somatic
- polygenic/complex genetic etiology.

These often result in a developmental abnormality or irreversible and progressive neuronal cell loss in the brain. Therefore, in these conditions, epilepsy is accompanied by other neurological deficits, such as ID, dementia or ataxia. Examples include inherited metabolic

TABLE 2.3

Examples of genes associated with epilepsy syndromes

Syndrome	Gene	Gene product
Self-limiting neonatal epilepsy	*KCNQ2* *KCNQ3*	Voltage-gated potassium channel subunits
Self-limiting familial neonatal-infantile seizures	*SCN2A*	Voltage-gated sodium channel, α subunit, type 2
Autosomal-dominant nocturnal frontal lobe epilepsy	*CHRNA4* *CHRNB2* *CHRNA2*	Nicotinic acetylcholine receptor subunits
Autosomal-dominant epilepsy with auditory features	*LGI1*	Leucine-rich glioma-inactivated protein
Genetic epilepsy with febrile seizures plus (GEFS+) and Dravet syndrome	*SCN1A, SCN1B* *SCN2A* *GABRG2*	Voltage-gated sodium channel subunits GABA$_A$ receptor, γ subunit, type 2
Severe myoclonic epilepsy of infancy	*SCN1A*	Voltage-gated sodium channel, α subunit, type 1

GABA, gamma-aminobutyric acid.

29

disorders, mitochondrial encephalopathies and neuronal migration disorders.

Metabolic disorders. Some metabolic disorders involve alteration of intracellular osmolarity. This causes biochemical changes leading to acute and severe electrolyte imbalance, such as hyponatremia, hypocalcemia and hypomagnesemia, resulting in seizures. In some cases, acute symptomatic seizures occur in individuals who do not have epilepsy. Replacing the missing chemical compound and regaining electrolyte balance may resolve the issue and not lead to a diagnosis of epilepsy. Most metabolic epilepsies are genetic in origin. Other unusual and complex metabolic disorders also have a genetic basis, such as GLUT1 deficiency syndrome in which the transportation of glucose to the brain is disturbed, resulting in brain damage and seizures.

Unknown etiology. Sometimes there is insufficient information to identify a cause for seizures.

Key points – classification and causes of seizures, epilepsy types and syndromes

- A seizure is a symptom of brain dysfunction.
- Depending on the pattern of onset, seizures are broadly classified into focal (partial) and generalized types; classification is important for identifying the underlying cause, prognosis and best approach to management.
- Minor seizures are often more important than major bilateral tonic–clonic seizures for an appropriate diagnosis, diagnostic tests and management strategies.
- Epileptic syndromes are defined by clinical features, aided by appropriate investigations that include EEG and brain imaging.
- Genetic mutations affecting ion channels have been identified in a range of rare idiopathic epilepsy syndromes.
- Etiology needs to be considered at every level and carries significant treatment implications.

Key references

1. Scheffer IE, Berkovic S, Capovilla G et al. ILAE classification of the epilepsies: position paper of the ILAE Commission for Classification and Terminology. *Epilepsia* 2017;58:512–21.

2. Fisher RS, Cross JH, French JA et al. Operational classification of seizure types by the International League Against Epilepsy: position paper of the ILAE Commission for Classification and Terminology. *Epilepsia* 2017;58:522–30.

3. Fisher RS, Cross JH, D'Souza C et al. Instruction manual for the ILAE 2017 operational classification of seizure types. *Epilepsia* 2017;58:531–42.

4. Brodie MJ, Zuberi SM, Scheffer IE et al. The 2017 ILAE classification of seizure types and the epilepsies: what do people with epilepsy and their caregivers need to know? *Epileptic Disord* 2018;20:77–87.

5. International League Against Epilepsy. *Diagnostic Manual.* International League Against Epilepsy, 2020. www.epilepsydiagnosis. org/?locale=en, last accessed 20 April 2022.

3 Diagnosis

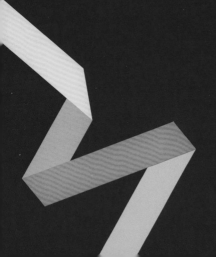

Epilepsy is not a single disease but an extensive collection of conditions with a wide range of underlying etiologies and pathologies, all sharing the common and fundamental characteristic of recurrent, usually unprovoked, seizures.[1] Chapter 2 describes the 2017 classification system for epilepsy, and this should be used to guide the diagnostic procedure.

When assessing an individual who presents with a seizure(s), three fundamental questions need to be addressed.
- Is/are the episode(s) epileptic seizure(s)?
- What is/are the seizure type(s)?
- What is the epilepsy syndrome?

When assessing a first-seizure patient for the first time, their age can guide the clinician toward a possible underlying etiology (Figure 3.1). For example, genetic epilepsies do not begin in people of pensionable age.

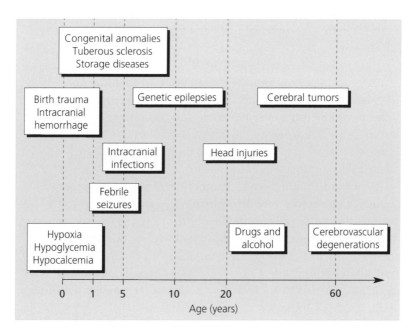

Figure 3.1 Etiology of epilepsy at different ages.

Clinical evaluation

Despite advances in investigative techniques, the diagnosis of epilepsy remains a clinical one.

History. A detailed history is the single most important step in the diagnostic process. When assessing a suspected first seizure, context is vital. Someone experiencing a seizure as part of an acute cerebral event may well not go on to develop epilepsy. These are known as acute symptomatic or provoked seizures and occur in close temporal relationship (often arbitrarily defined as within 1 week) with an acute insult of the CNS, which may be metabolic, toxic, structural, traumatic, infectious or inflammatory. Common examples include seizures during an acute stroke, encephalitis or electrolyte disturbance.

It has been estimated that up to 50% of all seizures may be acute symptomatic. Adequate effort should be made to search for any underlying acute CNS insult that may require urgent treatment. Unlike epileptic seizures, acute symptomatic seizures do not tend to recur. Therefore, as a general rule, long-term therapy with an ASM is not indicated for most individuals, although it may be warranted on a short-term basis until the acute condition is resolved.

The most important principle when assessing an individual with suspected seizures is for the clinician to visualize the event. Video recording using everyday devices, especially cell phones, has revolutionized clinicians' ability to see seizures. It is always advisable to ask if a seizure video has been taken, and to request a video of future events, particularly if the diagnosis is uncertain.

The patient should be carefully questioned about the suspected seizure. For instance, were there any obvious triggers? It is worth highlighting these early in the therapeutic relationship. The concept of life hygiene (see Chapter 6) and avoiding obvious seizure triggers can be crucial in the successful management of the condition and the mitigation of risk (Table 3.1).

Other questions to ask include: was there a warning for the seizure and how long did that last? Was consciousness lost or was awareness either partially or completely retained? How did the patient feel afterwards?

Clinicians should specifically ask about levels of confusion, using concrete examples: Did they recognize where they were or who they

TABLE 3.1

Seizure triggers

Common	Occasional
• Sleep deprivation	• Dehydration
• Alcohol withdrawal	• Barbiturate withdrawal
• Flickering lights (e.g. strobe lights, sunlight reflecting off water or through trees)	• Benzodiazepine withdrawal
	• Hyperventilation
• Proconvulsive drugs	• Flashing lights
• Systemic infection	• Dieting and missed meals
• Head trauma	• Specific 'reflex' triggers
• Recreational drugs	• Stress
• Non-adherence to ASM	• Intense exercise
• Menstruation	

were with? How long did the confusion last? Did they bite their tongue? If so, what part (lateral tongue bites are highly indicative of seizures due to epilepsy, whereas biting the tip has less association with epilepsy)?

Incontinence is not a reliable indicator for a seizure and can occur in other conditions involving paroxysmal events that can be mistaken for epilepsy.

Direct questioning about different seizure types can also be helpful (Table 3.2). The presence of other seizure types is crucial when identifying specific epilepsy syndromes, and thereby developing optimum treatment plans.

It is vital to obtain a witness history for the suspected seizure(s). Witnesses should be carefully questioned about the accuracy of the patient's account, particularly the timings of each stage of the seizure, before being asked what happened when (if) the patient lost awareness. Questions can be rephrased until a clear picture emerges of exactly what the seizure looked like. The following specific questions may be helpful.

• Did the jerking slow down toward the end of the seizure or stay the same?

TABLE 3.2

Helpful questions when eliciting seizure descriptions from patients or witnesses

Seizure types	Example questions
Myoclonic jerks (particularly in juvenile myoclonic epilepsy)	Does your cell phone fly out of your hand while checking overnight text messages?
	Do you drop your toothbrush while brushing your teeth in the morning?
Absences versus focal awareness-impaired seizures	Do you just realize that you have missed a sentence of conversation or were you unaware for a bit longer, say the length of an advert on TV or a pop song?
Focal awareness-impaired seizures	Does the person make repetitive movements, such as wringing their hands, rubbing their clothes or hair, chewing, swallowing or lip-smacking movements or sounds? (Indicative of temporal lobe involvement)
	Do they vocalize, or can they manage to form a simple word? (Useful for lateralization)
GTCS versus convulsive PNES	As the seizure progresses, do the jerks get bigger and slower or stay the same and stop suddenly?
	When the jerking stops, does the person stop breathing for a few seconds and then become deeply unaware for a short time, or do they recover quickly?
	How long after the seizure is it before they can talk and make sense?

- Did the seizure seem to start and stop?
- Were the patient's eyes open, closed, rolled back or deviated to one side?
- Did the patient exhibit any automatisms, such as swallowing, chewing, lip smacking or fiddling with their clothes?
- What was the patient like immediately after the seizure? Did the patient become deeply unresponsive? If so, for how long?
- How long did any confusion last and what was the level of the confusion?
- Did the patient need to sleep, or were they able to continue with the day's planned activities?

Physical examination is often unremarkable, although there may be focal neurological signs that correspond to an underlying structural abnormality in the brain. Investigations to identify underlying conditions that acutely provoke seizures should be guided by the clinical scenario. Routine blood tests should include full blood count and electrolytes, and an electrocardiogram (ECG) should be performed to detect cardiac arrhythmias and conduction abnormalities, particularly prolonged QT syndromes. Drug screening may be carried out when the history suggests drug abuse. Lumbar puncture for cerebrospinal fluid examination should be reserved for those suspected of having an acute CNS infection.

Cognitive evaluation is an important and sometimes neglected aspect of assessment. Arguably, this is more important in pediatrics, where cognitive decline associated with seizure onset may indicate an epileptic encephalopathy. In adults, epilepsy has cognitive implications, particularly around memory. This most often manifests as accelerated forgetting. The underlying etiology can be important: for example, traumatic brain injury or a cerebrovascular event will also, inevitably, cause some level of cognitive impairment.

Lifestyle considerations are clearly important, with alcohol presenting the triple whammy of cause, seizure trigger and cognitive impairment. It is important to recognize that seizures, particularly when prolonged, can cause significant cognitive decline, with convulsive SE leading to neuronal damage. Care should be taken when attributing cognitive or memory difficulties to a particular aspect of epilepsy management, particularly ASM, as the reasons are often multifactorial and diagnostic overshadowing can be a major problem.

Investigational technologies

Brain imaging (with MRI rather than CT where possible) and EEG are the primary investigations used in the diagnosis of epilepsy. Neither technology will confirm or refute a diagnosis of epilepsy and it is vital that the clinician understands when to request these tests, understands their uses and limitations and, crucially, poses the correct clinical questions.[2] It is important to provide the radiographer and/ or neurophysiologist with a detailed clinical history, including any response to treatment (if started), seizure descriptions and, if possible, a syndromic hypothesis.

Imaging should be requested in all instances of adult-onset epilepsy, unless it is possible to be certain that the epilepsy has a genetic cause. Imaging may identify the structural cause of focal epilepsies, but interictal EEGs can be normal in 50% of adults known to have epilepsy. Therefore, a diagnosis of epilepsy is not usually made from an EEG unless a seizure occurs during the recording. Even then, subtle focal aware seizures or seizures arising from the frontal lobe may not be detected. Conversely, a small number of people who have never experienced a seizure will have an epileptiform EEG.

Clinicians should not ask whether an EEG can confirm or refute the diagnosis of epilepsy, but whether it provides evidence for a particular epilepsy syndrome.[3] For example, it can be difficult to clinically differentiate primary generalized-onset from focal-onset tonic–clonic seizures. A confirmatory EEG in these circumstances may have a profound effect on the management of that individual. Recently, artificial intelligence (AI) has been used to analyze seizure video recordings of paroxysmal events during sleep. The system is not yet widely available, but it holds promise for people with relatively infrequent seizures or those who cannot tolerate EEG (for example, some people with ID).

Electroencephalography

Routine EEGs are often insensitive. Activation techniques, including hyperventilation and photic stimulation (Figure 3.2), are helpful in uncovering abnormalities. Diagnostic yield can also be increased by repeat recordings. If the initial EEG is unremarkable and the diagnosis remains in doubt, a sleep-deprivation study is recommended, particularly in the case of a suspected GGE, where it is mandated if the routine recording is non-contributory.

In a patient with suspected non-convulsive SE (see Chapter 7), an EEG can be diagnostic. An EEG can also immediately differentiate between epileptic and psychogenic non-epileptic convulsive SE.

In cases of a negative routine and/or sleep-deprived EEG, better detection of interictal and ictal events may be achieved with a prolonged EEG recording using portable equipment. On the plus side, this allows recording to take place in the patient's usual environment, but technical faults are more likely and accurate correlation with simultaneous behaviors on video is available only with certain recording systems. It also relies on the patient activating the camera, something that many patients fail to do.

Routine EEGs have a limited role in determining whether ASM can be safely tapered after a prolonged seizure-free interval; response to treatment and syndromic classification are more reliable indicators (see Chapter 4).

Structural imaging of the brain to look for underlying abnormalities is essential for the appropriate diagnostic evaluation of most patients with epilepsy, particularly those presenting with focal-onset seizures.[4] The imaging modality of choice is MRI. It has higher sensitivity

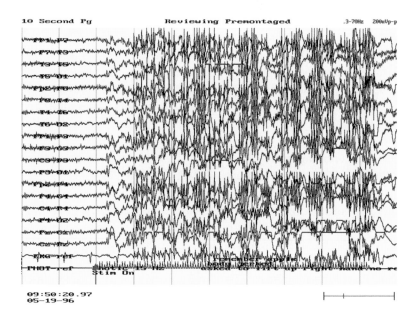

Figure 3.2 Photoconvulsive response provoked by intermittent photic stimulation. The arrow shows when photic stimulation began.

and specificity than CT for identifying structural lesions, such as malformations of cortical development (Figure 3.3a), hippocampal sclerosis, arteriovenous malformations, cavernous hemangioma (Figure 3.3b) and low-grade gliomas (Figure 3.3c). CT should be performed if MRI is unavailable and in patients for whom MRI is contraindicated (for example, those with cardiac pacemakers, non-compatible aneurysm clips or severe claustrophobia).

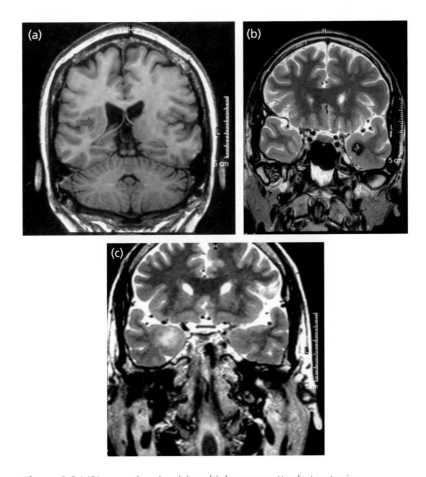

Figure 3.3 MRI scans showing (a) multiple grey matter heterotopia; (b) a cavernous hemangioma in the left temporal lobe; and (c) a low-grade glioma in the right temporal lobe.

Typical pathological findings vary with age. In young adults, frequently detected conditions are hippocampal sclerosis, sequelae of head trauma, congenital anomalies, brain tumors and vascular lesions. For patients in mid-life and beyond, scans are helpful in evaluating stroke and cerebral degeneration, and in identifying primary and secondary neoplasia.

Any patient with refractory epilepsy in whom the initial MRI scan is normal should have a high-resolution scan to exclude hippocampal atrophy and focal cortical dysplasia. The scan should be repeated periodically if there is one of the following:

- suspicion of a tumor
- worsening in the patient's neurological or cognitive function
- increase in the frequency or severity of the seizures.

Functional imaging can identify focal abnormalities in cerebral physiology, even when structural imaging results are normal. Single photon emission computed tomography (SPECT) can demonstrate increased blood flow in brain regions in association with seizure activity. Epileptogenic areas can be detected as hypometabolic regions interictally by PET (Figure 3.4). Magnetic resonance spectroscopy (MRS) can measure changes in chemical compounds in the brain associated with neuronal loss in certain epileptogenic pathologies. Functional neuroimaging techniques have a limited role in routine diagnostic evaluation, but they are useful adjuncts in the work-up for epilepsy surgery.[5]

Differential diagnoses

Several conditions can be mistaken for epilepsy (Table 3.3).[1] In adults, the commonest epilepsy imitators are syncopal events and PNES. The latter is particularly problematic (see Chapter 10).

Syncope (fainting) occurs when there is a sudden reduction in blood flow and oxygen supply to the brain, causing a transient loss of consciousness. Syncope has a lifetime prevalence of 40%, so it must always be suspected when investigating new-onset seizures.[6] Syncopal events can present with a simple collapse with rapid recovery, but may also include jerky movements, perhaps mistaken for myoclonus or even clonic or tonic–clonic seizures. Other people may look around

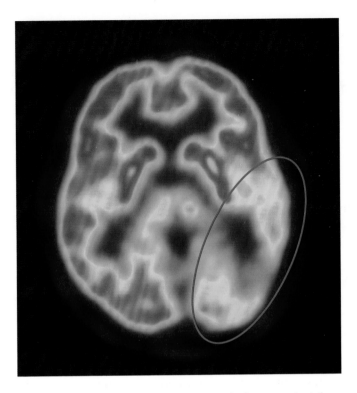

Figure 3.4 PET scan showing interictal hypometabolism over the left temporal and occipital areas (circled).

in a confused manner, mimicking a focal awareness-impaired seizure. Some people vocalize. Eyes are often open, again creating diagnostic difficulties.

The most common syncope is vasovagal. This can usually be identified by reliable triggers, such as getting up quickly or standing for prolonged periods, particularly in the context of peripheral vasodilation caused by a hot stuffy environment, crowded places, drug or alcohol use, frightening, emotional or unpleasant events and pain (medical procedures such as dentistry and phlebotomy are common precipitants). Warnings or auras usually occur. These include visual disturbance (classically, but not exclusively, loss of peripheral vision), feeling hot or clammy and becoming dizzy or unsteady. Cardiac

TABLE 3.3

Epilepsy imitators

Group	Examples in adults
Syncope and anoxic seizures	Vasovagal syncope
	Hyperventilation syncope
	Long QT and cardiac syncope
Behavioral, psychological and psychiatric disorders	Panic attacks
	Dissociative states
	PNES
Sleep-related conditions	Parasomnias
	Periodic leg movements
	Narcolepsy/cataplexy
Paroxysmal movement disorders	Tics
	Stereotypies
	Paroxysmal kinesigenic dyskinesia
Migraine-associated disorders	Migraine with visual aura
	Familial hemiplegic migraine
Miscellaneous events	Raised intracranial pressure

Adapted from ILAE 2020.[1]

syncope caused by cardiac arrhythmias or prolonged QT can also lead to cerebral hypoperfusion, often without the typical aura that occurs in vasovagal syncope. Cough and micturition syncope are relatively common and well recognized, the triggers being reflected in their names.

Key points – diagnosis

- Despite technological advances, the diagnosis of epilepsy remains a clinical one.
- Taking a detailed history is the single most important step in the diagnostic process.
- Visualizing a seizure via a video recording – including home recordings made on a cell phone – helps clinicians to assess individuals with suspected seizures.
- Careful questioning of patients and witnesses to a seizure can help to identify the type of seizure.
- Brain imaging and EEG cannot confirm or refute a diagnosis of epilepsy but can be used to look for underlying abnormalities and evidence of particular epilepsy syndromes.

References

1. International League Against Epilepsy. *Diagnostic Manual.* International League Against Epilepsy, 2020. www.epilepsydiagnosis.org, last accessed 20 April 2022.

2. Gaillard WD, Cross JH, Duncan JS et al. Epilepsy imaging study guideline criteria: commentary on diagnostic testing study guidelines and practice parameters. *Epilepsia* 2011;52,9:1750–6.

3. Tatum WO, Rubboli G, Kaplan PW et al. Clinical utility of EEG in diagnosing and monitoring epilepsy in adults. *Clin Neurophysiol* 2018;129,5:1056–82.

4. Sone D. Making the invisible visible: advanced neuroimaging techniques in focal epilepsy. *Front Neurosci* 2021;15:699176.

5. Algahtany M, Abdrabou A, Elhaddad A, Alghamdi A. Advances in brain imaging techniques for patients with intractable epilepsy. *Front Neurosci* 2021;15:699123.

6. Hackethal V. Epilepsy, syncope, or both? NeurologyLive, 2017. www.neurologylive.com/view/epilepsy-syncope-or-both, last accessed 20 April 2022.

Further reading

National Institute for Health and Care Excellence (NICE). *Epilepsies in Children, Young People and Adults. NICE guideline [NG217].* NICE, 2022. www.nice.org.uk/guidance/ng217, last accessed 6 June 2022.

Scottish Intercollegiate Guidelines Network (SIGN). SIGN 143. Diagnosis and Management of Epilepsy in Adults. SIGN, 2018. www.sign.ac.uk/media/1079/sign143_2018.pdf

4 Pharmacological management

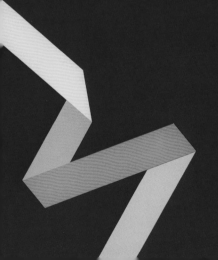

HEALTHCARE

Starting treatment

Several questions need to be addressed when deciding whether to prescribe an ASM to an individual presenting after one or more seizures.

- What is the relative risk of recurrence?
- What are the potential negative consequences on the patient's life if seizures recur?
- What are the potential adverse effects of treatment?

After a single seizure. Treatment should be considered after the first tonic–clonic seizure when the risk of recurrence is high, for instance, if there is an underlying cerebral lesion, abnormal EEG or strong family history of epilepsy, or if the individual has previously experienced myoclonic, absence or focal seizures. In some instances, the patient may wish to start treatment after a single event because they are concerned about the potentially significant impact that recurrent seizures could have on their lifestyle, such as their ability to legally drive a car.[1] A systematic review of etiologies identified a 66.6% risk of recurrence after first seizure following stroke, traumatic brain injury, cerebral lesions and unspecified CNS infections.[2] In the absence of these etiologies, recurrence risk after a first seizure is about 50%, rising to over 70% after a second event.

After more than one seizure. Patients reporting more than one well-documented or witnessed seizure require treatment. Exceptions can include widely separated seizures or provoked seizures, for which specific treatments or avoidance activity (see Chapter 6) may be sufficient prophylaxis (for example, concomitant illness such as infection or metabolic disturbance, photosensitive epilepsy, alcohol withdrawal). In addition, treatment is unlikely to succeed in patients unlikely or unwilling to take medication as prescribed (such as some alcohol abusers or drug addicts, or people who refuse to take medication on principle).

The decision to start treatment should be made after a full discussion of the risks and benefits with the patient and their family. The information should be presented in the context of what is known and what is conjecture about the risk of recurrent seizures, the chance of a successful outcome with treatment and the likelihood of remission. Pushing the issue if there is doubt about the diagnosis, particularly if the patient resists the introduction of ASM, may be counterproductive. Ideally, the patient and their immediate family should be encouraged to make an informed commitment to the treatment plan.[1,3]

Reasons for taking prophylactic treatment should be discussed at the outset. When prescribing an ASM, the clinician must also discuss all common side effects, as well as uncommon but serious drug-related problems such as the risk of teratogenesis in women of childbearing potential. That this particular risk has been touched upon should be documented in the patient's case notes. Similarly, the regulations regarding driving should be raised and documented. Time should be taken to deal with the patient's fears, misconceptions and prejudices, as well as those of the family. The importance of total adherence to medication should also be stressed. These issues often require further emphasis at subsequent visits.

The possibility of SUDEP and safety issues should be thoroughly discussed at the point of diagnosis, as well as at subsequent consultations, especially if adherence is an issue or if seizures remain uncontrolled. The provision of written material can be a useful way to ensure that nothing important is overlooked.[1,3]

Principles of drug selection

The goal of treatment should be to enable the patient to lead as normal a lifestyle as possible, which generally requires complete seizure control without, or with minimal, side effects. Choosing the most suitable ASM requires knowledge of the epilepsy characteristics, the individual and the available drugs (see Chapter 5). The issues discussed below should be included in the decision-making process.

Monotherapy is associated with better adherence and fewer side effects than combination therapy. It is also likely to be more cost-effective. For these reasons, in general, serial monotherapy trials of two appropriate first-line drugs can be tried before combinations. The chance of remission is highest with the first ASM (Figure 4.1): a 30-year longitudinal cohort study reported that 86.8% of people with epilepsy who had achieved 1-year seizure control were on monotherapy and 89.9% achieved seizure control with the first or second ASM.[4] Substantial attention should therefore be given to choosing the most appropriate initial ASM, taking into account a range of factors, including the seizure type(s) and/or epilepsy syndrome. Other relevant issues include age, sex, weight, psychiatric and other comorbidities, childbearing potential and concomitant medication.[4]

Efficacy and tolerability. ASM effectiveness is a function of efficacy and tolerability. Given that lifelong treatment is often required, even in patients with mild epilepsy, safety and lack of long-term sequelae are also important considerations when selecting treatment.

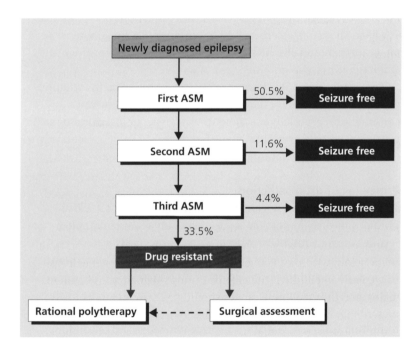

Figure 4.1 Strategies for managing newly diagnosed epilepsy. Of 906 patients, 50.5% remained seizure free for 1 year or longer with the initial ASM (monotherapy). If this failed, the second and third regimens (monotherapy or combination therapy) provided an additional 11.6% and 4.4% likelihood of seizure freedom, respectively. Adapted from data in Chen et al. 2018.[4]

Titration and monitoring. Approximately 50% of newly diagnosed patients will be able to tolerate and become seizure free with the first ASM, often at low or moderate doses.[4] In general, ASM should be started at a low dose, with increments over several weeks to establish an effective and tolerable regimen. Some agents, such as sodium valproate (VPA) and levetiracetam (LEV), can be commenced at effective doses with, or even without, a rapid titration phase. Slow titration will help avoid concentration-dependent side effects, as experienced with carbamazepine (CBZ) or topiramate (TPM), in particular CNS toxicity, which is likely to discourage the patient from persevering with therapy in the long term.

An additional benefit of a cautious approach is that it allows tolerance to sedation or cognitive impairment to develop. Such a policy will also ensure early detection of potentially serious idiosyncratic reactions, such as rash, hepatotoxicity and blood dyscrasias.[5] Slow titration with lamotrigine (LTG) has been shown to reduce the risk of skin rash.[1,5] Neurotoxicity typically occurs with higher doses of ASM, and a gradual titration policy may allow seizure freedom to be recognized at lower doses, thus aiding safety and adherence.

Measuring serum ASM concentrations can help to determine the extent of adherence, assess side effects and establish the most effective dose for a seizure-free patient. Concentrations should be measured each time a patient with established epilepsy is admitted acutely for seizures. Serum ASM concentrations associated with optimal control or with neurotoxicity vary from patient to patient and may occur below, within or above the therapeutic ranges for the drugs, particularly in children, the elderly, during pregnancy and patients taking polytherapy. These ranges should be regarded as a guide to prescribing. Routine measurement of serum levels of newer ASM is not otherwise recommended, as they do not correlate well on a population basis with efficacy or side effects.[6]

Measurement of free serum phenytoin (PHT) concentrations can occasionally be useful when patients have low serum albumin levels or take other medications that bind tightly to protein. PHT is probably the only ASM for which regular (annual) measurements are useful. Women who experience exacerbation of seizures just before their menses should have serum ASM concentrations checked in the premenstrual period and compared with mid-cycle concentrations, as levels can drop markedly just before and during menstruation. This can be a particular problem with LTG. Altering ASM dose during the menstrual cycle is problematic as there is a delay in achieving steady state levels. However, intermittent clobazam (CLB), started a few days before levels are predicted to fall, can be a helpful strategy.

If the first drug is well tolerated but the seizures persist, the dose should be increased toward the limit of tolerability, aiming for complete seizure freedom. If the first ASM produces an idiosyncratic reaction or side effects at low or moderate doses, or fails to improve seizure control, an alternative drug should be substituted.[1,3]

First-line ASM treatment options

Focal-onset epilepsy. LTG has been found to be more effective and better tolerated long term than CBZ, TPM and oxcarbazepine (OXC).[1,3,7] LEV and zonisamide (ZNS) are also used in monotherapy,[1,3,5] though may be less effective than LTG.[1,3,7]

Generalized-onset epilepsy. VPA is clinically more effective and cost-effective than LTG and LEV.[7] However, VPA is not recommended for girls and women of child-bearing age because of a high risk of teratogenicity (see Chapter 8). Ethosuximide (ESM) and VPA are both effective in controlling absences, while VPA, ZNS, LEV TPM, clonazepam (CZP) and, to a lesser extent, LTG can be useful for myoclonic jerks.[7]

Matching treatment to seizure type. The profile of activity against different seizure types differs among different ASM (Table 4.1). Some epilepsy syndromes have been found to be particularly responsive to specific therapeutic agents. For instance, juvenile myoclonic epilepsy (which is a lifelong condition) responds well to VPA. On the other hand, myoclonic and absence seizures can be exacerbated by PHT, CBZ, gabapentin (GBP), pregabalin (PGB), OXC, tiagabine (TGB), eslicarbazepine acetate (ESL) and vigabatrin (VGB). It is therefore of paramount importance to classify the patient's seizure type(s) and epilepsy syndrome accurately (see Chapter 2). The recommended drug choices in Table 4.1 are based on the current literature and UK and US treatment guidelines. Because of the paucity of head-to-head

TABLE 4.1

Efficacy of ASM against common seizure types and syndromes

		Type of seizure/syndrome				
ASM	Focal	Focal to bilateral tonic–clonic	Tonic–clonic	Absence	Myoclonic	Lennox–Gastaut
BRV	+	+	+	?	+	?
CBZ	+	+	+	–	–	0
CEN	+	+	?	?	?	?
CLB	+	+	+	?	+	+
CZP	+	+	+	?	+	?+
ESL	+	+	+	–	–	0
ESM	0	0	0	+	0	0
FBM	+	+	?+	?+	?	+
GBP	+	+	?	–	–	?
LCM	+	+	+	?	?	?
LEV	+	+	+	?	+	?
LTG	+	+	+	+	+*	+
OXC	+	+	+	–	–	0
PB	+	+	+	0	?+	?
PER	+	+	?	?	?	?
PGB	+	+	?	–	–	?
PHT	+	+	+	–	–	0
PRM	+	+	+	0	?	?
RFN	+	+	+	+	?	+
TGB	+	+	?	–	?	?
TPM	+	+	+	?	+	+
VGB	+	+	?	–	–	?
VPA	+	+	+	+	+	+
ZNS	+	+	+	?+	+	?+

*Lamotrigine may worsen myoclonic seizures in some cases. + proven efficacy;
?+ probable efficacy; 0 ineffective; – worsens control; ? unknown.
BRV, brivaracetam; CBZ, carbamazepine; CEN, cenobamate; CLB, clobazam;
CZP, clonazepam; ESL, eslicarbazepine acetate; ESM, ethosuximide; FBM, felbamate;
GBP, gabapentin; LCM, lacosamide; LEV, levetiracetam; LTG, lamotrigine;
OXC, oxcarbazepine; PB, phenobarbital; PER, perampanel; PGB, pregabalin;
PHT, phenytoin; PRM, primidone; RFN, rufinamide; TGB, tiagabine; TPM, topiramate;
VGB, vigabatrin; VPA, sodium valproate; ZNS, zonisamide.

comparative studies, particularly for newer ASM, the evidence base is supplemented by the authors' personal experience.

Side effects

Safety concerns include idiosyncratic reactions, long-term complications and teratogenicity. The most common idiosyncratic reaction is skin rash, which affects up to 10% of patients taking CBZ, PHT or LTG and usually resolves once the ASM has been withdrawn.[1] Severe life-threatening cutaneous reactions (Stevens–Johnson syndrome or toxic epidermal necrolysis) and drug reaction with eosinophilia and systemic symptoms (DRESS) may occur in patients taking LTG, usually within a few weeks of initiating treatment.[1] Genetic testing is recommended in Asian, Japanese and European populations before commencing CBZ (and PHT, ESL and OXC) because of an increased risk of developing severe cutaneous reactions (see Chapter 5).

Hypersensitivity syndrome (fever, rash, lymphadenopathy and multiorgan failure) associated with ASM can occur in up to 5 in 10 000 people within 8 weeks of initiating treatment and treatment should be stopped immediately.[1]

Suicidal thoughts and changes in mood and behavior are a potential side effect of most ASM.[1,3,5] Clinicians should monitor patients for changes in mental health status, and patients should be encouraged to discuss worsening symptoms with their clinicians.[1] When there is a history of previous suicidal ideation, LEV, TPM and GBP should be avoided. These drugs should be used with caution in those with psychiatric illness such as depression.[1,3,8] TPM, TGB, VGB and ZNS may worsen psychosis[1,8]. Other considerations are the potential negative effects on behavior and cognition (Table 4.2).[1,3,5]

Rare cases of acute glaucoma, increased risk of renal calculi (kidney stones) and clinically important hypohydrosis (sweating) can complicate TPM administration; renal calculi and hypohydrosis have also been reported for ZNS,[3,5] and concomitant use should be avoided.

Long-term use of some ASM can lead to specific side effects (see Chapter 5) including dysmorphic changes, such as gum hypertrophy with PHT and weight gain with VPA, GBP and PGB. TPM and ZNS, on the other hand, often produce weight loss. The high

TABLE 4.2

Adverse effects of ASM on cognition and behavior

ASM	Cognitive	Behavioral
BRV	0	+?
CBZ	+	0
CEN	0	0
CLB	+	+
CZP	++	+
ESL	0	0
ESM	+	+
FBM	0	+
GBP	0	0
LCM	0	0
LEV	0	++
LTG	0	0
OXC	+?	0
PB	++	++
PER	0	+*
PGB	0	0
PHT	+	0
PRM	++	++
RFN	0	0
TGB	0	0
TPM	+*	+
VGB	0	+
VPA	+	0
ZNS	0	+

*Risk reduced by slow titration. ^ limited real world data; 0 no effect;
+? possible effect; + mild effect; ++ marked effect.
BRV, brivaracetam; CBZ, carbamazepine; CEN, cenobamate; CLB, clobazam;
CZP, clonazepam; ESL, eslicarbazepine acetate; ESM, ethosuximide; FBM, felbamate;
GBP, gabapentin; LCM, lacosamide; LEV, levetiracetam; LTG, lamotrigine;
OXC, oxcarbazepine; PB, phenobarbital; PER, perampanel; PGB, pregabalin;
PHT, phenytoin; PRM, primidone; RFN, rufinamide; TGB, tiagabine; TPM, topiramate;
VGB, vigabatrin; VPA, sodium valproate; ZNS, zonisamide.

incidence of concentric visual field defects in patients receiving VGB has substantially reduced the clinical use of this otherwise effective agent.

The teratogenic risks associated with ASM are discussed in Chapter 8. Girls and women of child-bearing age should only be treated with VPA if it is the only ASM that will adequately control their seizures. VPA can also be associated with polycystic ovary syndrome and hyperinsulinemia in susceptible women.[5]

Pharmacokinetics and drug–drug interactions

Pharmacokinetic interactions affect the absorption, distribution or elimination of ASM while pharmacodynamic interactions refer to synergism and antagonism of ASM at the site of action.[9] An ideal ASM should demonstrate complete absorption, linear kinetics and a long elimination half-life, allowing once- or twice-daily dosing. Low protein binding, lack of active metabolites and clearance by the renal route can also be regarded as advantageous, as a drug with these characteristics is likely to be easy to use and less likely to be implicated in pharmacokinetic interactions. However, the dose for drugs that are excreted unchanged by the kidney, such as GBP and PGB, will need to be adjusted in patients with renal impairment in relation to creatinine clearance.

Enzyme-inducing ASM are notorious for their pharmacodynamic interactions with each other and with other medications via their effect on the hepatic cytochrome P450 (CYP450) enzyme system (Table 4.3). Phenobarbital (PB), primidone (PRM), PHT, OXC, ESL, TPM and CBZ induce CYP450 enzymes that accelerate the breakdown of many commonly prescribed lipid-soluble drugs metabolized by the same system, including oral contraceptives, cytotoxics, antiretrovirals, cardiac antiarrhythmics, immunosuppressants and warfarin. VPA is a weak CYP450 enzyme inhibitor, and as such can slow the clearance of other ASM such as PHT and LTG. ASM can also be a target for other drugs that induce or inhibit hepatic metabolism. Newer ASM are less likely to interfere with hepatic metabolism, although OXC, felbamate (FBM), rufinamide (RFN), ESL at doses above 800 mg daily and TPM at daily doses above 200 mg selectively induce the breakdown of the estrogenic component of the oral contraceptive pill (OCP).[1,9]

TABLE 4.3

Pharmacokinetic characteristics of ASM

	Undergoes hepatic metabolism	Affects drug-metabolizing enzymes	Associated with ASM interactions
BRV	No	No	No
CBZ	Yes	Yes	Yes
CEN	Yes	Yes	Yes
CLB	Yes	No	Yes
CZP	Yes	No	Yes
ESL	Yes	Yes	Yes
ESM	Yes	No	Yes
FBM	Yes	Yes	Yes
GBP	No	No	No
LCM	Yes	No	No
LEV	No	No	No
LTG	Yes	No	Yes
OXC	Yes	Yes	Yes
PB	Yes	Yes	Yes
PER	Yes	No	Yes
PGB	No	No	No
PHT	Yes	Yes	Yes
PRM	Yes	Yes	Yes
RFN	Yes	Yes	Yes
TGB	Yes	No	Yes
TPM	Yes	Yes	Yes
VGB	No	No	Yes
VPA	Yes	Yes	Yes
ZNS	Yes	No	Yes

BRV, brivaracetam; CBZ, carbamazepine; CEN, cenobamate; CLB, clobazam; CZP, clonazepam; ESL, eslicarbazepine acetate; ESM, ethosuximide; FBM, felbamate; GBP, gabapentin; LCM, lacosamide; LEV, levetiracetam; LTG, lamotrigine; OXC, oxcarbazepine; PB, phenobarbital; PER, perampanel; PGB, pregabalin; PHT, phenytoin; PRM, primidone; RFN, rufinamide; TGB, tiagabine; TPM, topiramate; VGB, vigabatrin; VPA, sodium valproate; ZNS, zonisamide.

Comorbidities

As well as controlling seizures, some ASM have demonstrated efficacy for the treatment of other conditions that may coexist with epilepsy (Table 4.4). For instance, VPA has traditionally been used in bipolar disorder.[5] It is also effective prophylaxis for migraine, an indication for which TPM has also been approved.[5] GBP is effective for the treatment of certain neuropathic pain syndromes, while PGB has demonstrated efficacy for neuropathic pain and generalized anxiety disorder.[5] LTG has been licensed for bipolar disorder.[5] With a widening spectrum of indications, ASM selection may be tailored according to the patient's neurological and psychiatric comorbidities (see Chapter 9).

Bone health

Long-term ASM treatment can lead to hypocalcemia and decrease biologically active vitamin D levels, resulting in reduced bone mineral density (BMD) and higher risk of fractures. A long-term study of people with epilepsy treated with ASM found that bone density did not worsen in 79% of patients, while 21% developed new osteopenia or osteoporosis.[10] Risk factors for abnormal BMD include age, dose

TABLE 4.4

ASM with efficacy in non-epileptic conditions*

Neuropathic pain	Migraine prophylaxis	Essential tremor	Anxiety	Bipolar disorder
CBZ	VPA	PRM	GBP	CBZ
OXC	TPM	TPM	PGB	OXC
LTG			CLB	VPA
GBP				LTG
PGB				
LCM				

*Indications for non-epileptic conditions vary among different countries.
CBZ, carbamazepine; CLB, clobazam; GBP, gabapentin; LCM, lacosamide; LEV, levetiracetam; LTG, lamotrigine; OXC, oxcarbazepine; PGB, pregabalin; PHT, phenytoin; PRM, primidone; TPM, topiramate; VPA, sodium valproate.

and increased duration of ASM treatment, polytherapy, coexisting comorbidities, body mass index, menopause and other factors such as poor nutrition, inadequate sunlight and immobility.[10,11] Both enzyme-inducing (such as CBZ, PHT, PB) and non-enzyme-inducing ASM (such as VPA) are implicated, and the effects may be additive. Evidence for newer ASM affecting bone health is limited. There are a variety of mechanisms for ASM-induced bone abnormalities, the most important of which appears to be an increased rate of bone turnover. Bone loss can be detected by dual-energy X-ray absorptiometry (DEXA) or quantitative ultrasound.[11]

To minimize the risk of reduced BMD, patients receiving long-term ASM treatment are advised to maintain the optimal level of physical activity, a balanced diet and exposure to sunshine. Calcium and vitamin D supplements are recommended, as well as regular DEXA scans. Patients should be encouraged to stop smoking and reduce alcohol intake.[10,11] To reduce fracture risk, strategies should be put in place to prevent falls in patients experiencing seizures.[12] Once osteopenia or osteoporosis has developed, the patient should be referred to an endocrinologist for appropriate therapy.

Drug-resistant epilepsy

Despite the introduction of many new ASM over the last 30 years, the rate of drug-resistant epilepsy remains stubbornly high at around 30%. Chapter 6 discusses non-pharmacological options for this cohort of people. Nevertheless, the majority will still be treated with ASM. Studies have shown that careful and systematic review of medication and the logical selection of additional ASM can result in significant seizure improvement, and for some people even seizure freedom, disproving the nihilistic view that intractability is inevitable if seizure control is not obtained rapidly after therapy is started.[12]

Individuals who fail to adequately respond to initial therapy should be reassessed before additional ASM is considered. A proportion will have pseudoresistant epilepsy. There can be several reasons for this, including incorrect diagnosis, incorrect classification of epilepsy, poor treatment adherence, ongoing seizure triggers and poor choice of ASM (Table 4.5). Assuming the diagnosis is correct, a careful review of the patient's existing ASM should be undertaken, including drugs that may have been tried in the past and subsequently withdrawn. It is possible that this review will result in a reasonable monotherapy option. However, most people who have failed to achieve seizure freedom with the first two medications will require polytherapy.[13]

Predicting which patients may become resistant is difficult, but it is important to do so given that their risk of SUDEP, and other causes of mortality, is much greater than for those with well-controlled seizures. The intrinsic neurobiological pattern underlying the epilepsy in syndromes such as Lennox–Gastaut (LGS) and Dravet (DS) make drug resistance the rule rather than the exception. Other risk factors are young age of onset (less than 1 year), abnormal neuroimaging, etiology, concomitant neuropsychiatric disorders or ID, prolonged febrile seizures or SE, a large number of seizures in the year before starting treatment, previous drug misuse, epilepsy in first-degree relatives and specific EEG abnormalities.[4] An inadequate response to initial ASM treatment is also prognostic.

TABLE 4.5

Some reasons for pseudoresistance to ASM

Wrong diagnosis

- Syncope, cardiac arrhythmia, for example
- PNES (see Chapter 10)
- Underlying brain neoplasm

Wrong drug(s)

- Inappropriate for seizure type
- Pharmacokinetic/pharmacodynamic interactions

Wrong dose

- Too low (if target range is ignored)
- Side effects preventing dose increase

Wrong lifestyle

- Poor adherence with medication
- Inappropriate choices (e.g. alcohol or drug abuse)

Rational polypharmacy

Prior to the 1970s, polytherapy was commonplace, with drugs such as PB and PHT often being given concurrently as first-choice treatment. Studies during the following two decades suggested that monotherapy was at least as effective in terms of controlling seizures and was generally better tolerated. This is still the view in terms of initial treatment. However, in drug-resistant epilepsy so-called rational polytherapy is now considered the best approach. General management principles (Table 4.6) are just as true for polytherapy as monotherapy. However, there are important additional considerations.

As discussed above, pharmacodynamic and pharmacokinetic interactions between ASM are common. This is not necessarily all bad.

TABLE 4.6

Ten commandments in the pharmacological treatment of epilepsy

- Choose the correct drug for the seizure type and/or epilepsy syndrome
- Start at a low dose unless the patient is having frequent seizures
- Titrate up slowly to allow the development of tolerance to CNS side effects
- Keep the regimen simple with once- or twice-daily dosing if possible
- Measure drug concentration to monitor adherence and to correlate with later seizure control and side effects
- Counsel the patient early regarding the implications of the diagnosis, the prophylactic nature of drug therapy, the importance of absolute adherence and the risk of SUDEP
- Try two reasonable ASM as monotherapy before adding a second drug in combination
- When seizures persist, combine the best-tolerated first-line drug with one of the newer agents, depending on seizure type and mechanisms of action
- Simplify medication schedules and regimens as much as possible in patients receiving polypharmacy
- Aim for the best seizure control consistent with optimal quality of life in patients with drug-resistant epilepsy

Some combinations have been shown to have synergistic properties, the best documented being between VPA and LTG (Table 4.7).[14] The paucity of further well-constructed trials of combination therapy is surprising, given the number of people requiring this approach. Much of the additional evidence has been observational, based on preclinical studies uncovering trends when a new ASM is added to existing therapy. Interactions can also significantly limit dosage and may even preclude the use of certain combinations. ZNS and TPM when given together have an unacceptably high risk of renal calculi. VPA and LTG need very cautious titration when one is added to the other, because of the increased risk of serious hypersensitivity reactions. The maximum dose will also be limited because of increased neurotoxicity. Drugs with less favorable neurocognitive and/or neurobehavioral side effects will require careful monitoring if used in combination (see Table 4.2).

Combining ASM with different modes of action is important.[13] For example, it is better to combine a sodium channel-blocking drug with an agent that exerts its primary mode of action by binding to the synaptic vesicle glycoprotein 2A (SV2A) (such as LAC and LEV or CBZ and LEV) or enhances the effects of gamma-aminobutyric

TABLE 4.7

Useful ASM combinations

Combination	Indication
VPA and ESM	Generalized absences
CBZ and VPA	Focal onset seizures
VPA and LTG*	Focal/generalized seizures
TPM and LTG	Focal/generalized seizures
VPA and LEV	Focal/generalized seizures
LTG and LEV	Focal/generalized seizures
LEV and LCM	Focal/generalized seizures

*This is the only combination for which good laboratory and clinical evidence exists in support of synergism.

CBZ, carbamazepine; ESM, ethosuximide; LCM, lacosamide; LEV, levetiracetam; LTG, lamotrigine; TPM, topiramate; VPA, sodium valproate.

acid (GABA) (such as LTG and VPA) than to use sodium channel blockers in combination. However, there are caveats to this principle. For example, LTG and ESL may be effective because the former enhances fast inactivation of voltage-gated sodium channels, whereas the latter enhances slow inactivation. Conversely, LTG and CBZ both affect sodium channels in the same way. That, coupled with a significant pharmacokinetic interaction that will significantly reduce LTG levels,[15] makes this combination particularly undesirable.

ASM withdrawal

Successful treatment outcome can be regarded as freedom from seizures without side effects. Individuals most likely to remain seizure free are those who have relatively few seizures before and after starting ASM therapy, those treated with a single ASM and those who have been seizure free for many years. Individuals in whom treatment is successful are more likely to lead rewarding lives than those with uncontrolled seizures, with optimal intellectual and emotional development and positive educational and vocational achievements. Eventually, some patients can have their medication withdrawn and remain in remission.

Patients who are 'doing well' may want to stop treatment for a variety of reasons, including the awareness of side effects or the subjective perception of subtle deterioration in cognitive function. Some people do not equate taking medication with normal health. Finally, the person may want to start a family and may be concerned about the possible negative effects of ASM on reproductive function, along with the specter of teratogenesis.

Conversely, some patients with a high chance of successful ASM withdrawal may choose to stay on drugs in the long term, because of fear of further seizures or for practical reasons, such as driving (in most jurisdictions driving must cease while ASM withdrawal is attempted and for a period after the drug has been stopped, even if seizures do not occur). The decision to withdraw ASM should therefore only be made after careful discussion between the patient and an epilepsy specialist. It should never be undertaken by the patient themselves or by a general practitioner.[3]

Several studies have shown that after a long period of perfect seizure control, medication can be stopped without seizure recurrence (for several years at least) in around 60% of patients. There are no data to guide the length of the seizure-free period but a flexible 5-year seizure-free period is considered prudent in adults. A mathematical model was developed in 1993 to predict outcomes following ASM withdrawal.[16] Important factors in favor of successful withdrawal are seizure freedom using one ASM, no seizures after starting ASM treatment, several years of seizure freedom (5 years is optimal), no history of myoclonic or tonic–clonic seizures and a normal EEG.

Seizure type or epilepsy syndrome is not absolutely predictive of recurrence. Some forms of idiopathic generalized seizures, either absence or tonic–clonic, are less likely to recur once they are under control. Even complex partial seizures can disappear after a long period of freedom from seizures. EEG is not a huge help in predicting seizure recurrence, but it can be reassuring if undertaken before starting withdrawal, part way through and shortly after withdrawal is complete, particularly for patients with IGEs.

There are no standard protocols for optimal tapering of medication. Most specialists advise slow reduction by decrements over at least 6 months. As a rule of thumb, the longer the patient has taken an ASM, the longer the downward titration should take. If the patient is being treated with two types of ASM, one drug should be slowly withdrawn before the second is tapered. More than 90% of recurrences will occur during the year following withdrawal, and many will present during or shortly after the tapering period.[17]

Key points – pharmacological management

- Patients reporting more than one unprovoked seizure usually require treatment; treatment after a single unprovoked seizure could be considered if the chance of recurrence is high.
- At the start of treatment, a single ASM should be given at a low dose and slowly titrated to an effective dose.
- First-line ASM should be chosen according to the patient's seizure type(s) and/or epilepsy syndrome. Other important factors include the likelihood of side effects, lack of long-term sequelae and a low potential for pharmacokinetic interactions.
- Combinations of ASM should be used after failure of two monotherapies in series, or if the first ASM is well tolerated but fails to completely control the seizures.
- Drug-resistant epilepsy is defined as the failure of two tolerated and appropriate types of ASM (whether as monotherapies or in combination) to achieve sustained seizure freedom.
- A small number of patients will demonstrate a sustained response to the fourth, fifth, sixth or even seventh ASM and so drug-resistant epilepsy should never be viewed nihilistically.
- None of the newer ASM has shown superior efficacy when tested against established agents for the treatment of focal seizures and GTCS, although some may be better tolerated.
- Patients should be referred to a specialist for definitive diagnosis and initiation of treatment, or when seizures prove resistant to medication, they are planning for pregnancy or hoping to stop treatment in the case of remission.
- The patient should have a named point of contact to help them with the management of their epilepsy, which could be an epilepsy specialist nurse, neurologist or primary care physician (who is usually vital in terms of repeat prescriptions).

References

1. Scottish Intercollegiate Guidelines Network. Diagnosis and management of epilepsy in adults: a national clinical guideline. Scottish Intercollegiate Guidelines Network, 2018. www.sign.ac.uk/media/1079/sign143_2018.pdf, last accessed 20 February 2022.

2. López SV, Ramos-Jiménez C, de la Cruz Reyes LA et al. Epilepsy diagnosis based on one unprovoked seizure and ≥60% risk. A systematic review of the etiologies. *Epilepsy Behav* 2021;125:108392.

3. National Institute for Health and Care Excellence (NICE). *Epilepsies in Children, Young People and Adults. NICE guideline [NG217]*. National Institute for Health and Care Excellence, 2022. www.nice.org.uk/guidance/ng217, last accessed 6 June 2022.

4. Chen Z, Brodie MJ, Liew D, Kwan P. Treatment outcomes in patients with newly diagnosed epilepsy treated with established and new antiepileptic drugs: a 30-year longitudinal cohort study. *JAMA Neurol* 2018;75:279–86.

5. National Institute for Health and Care Excellence (NICE). *Epilepsy*. NICE, 2022. bnf.nice.org.uk/treatment-summary/epilepsy.html, last accessed 22 February 2022.

6. Landmark SJ, Johannessen SI, Patsalos PN. Therapeutic drug monitoring of antiepileptic drugs: current status and future prospects. *Expert Opin Drug Metab Toxicol* 2020;16:227–38.

7. Marson A, Burnside G, Appleton R et al. The SANAD II study of the effectiveness and cost-effectiveness of valproate versus levetiracetam for newly diagnosed generalised and unclassifiable epilepsy: an open-label, non-inferiority, multicentre, phase 4, randomised controlled trial. *Lancet* 2021;397:1375–86.

8. Srinivas HV, Shah U. Comorbidities of epilepsy. *Neurol India* 2017;65:S18–24.

9. Zaccara G, Perucca E. Interactions between antiepileptic drugs, and between antiepileptic drugs and other drugs. *Epileptic Disord* 2014;16:409–31.

10. Miller AS, Ferastraoaru V, Tabatabaie V et al. Are we responding effectively to bone mineral density loss and fracture risks in people with epilepsy? *Epilepsia Open* 2020;5:240–7.

11. Arora E, Singh H, Gupta YK. Impact of antiepileptic drugs on bone health: need for monitoring, treatment, and prevention strategies. *J Fam Med Prim Care* 2016;5:248–53.

12. Luciano AL, Shorvon SD. Results of treatment changes in patients with apparently drug-resistant chronic epilepsy. *Ann Neurol* 2007;62:375–81.

13. Fattorusso A, Matricardi S, Mencaroni E et al. The pharmacoresistant epilepsy: an overview on existant and new emerging therapies. *Front Neurol* 2021;12:674483.

14. Brodie MJ, Yuen AW. Lamotrigine substitution study: evidence for synergism with sodium valproate? 105 study group. *Epilepsy Res* 1997;26:423–32.

15. Pastalos PN. *Antiepileptic Drug Interactions: A Clinical Guide.* Clarius Press, 2005.

16. Medical Research Council Antiepileptic Drug Withdrawal Study Group. Prognostic index for recurrence of seizures after remission of epilepsy. *BMJ* 1993;306:1374–8.

17. Medical Research Council Antiepileptic Drug Withdrawal Study Group. Randomised study of antiepileptic drug withdrawal in patients in remission. *Lancet* 1991;337:1175–80.

Neurology and
Neuroscience

5 Antiseizure medications

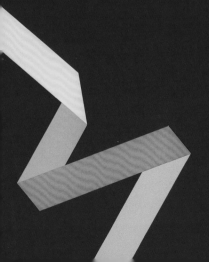

HEALTHCARE

This chapter provides a quick reference to the main characteristics of approved ASM, including indications, mechanisms of action, contraindications, side effects and significant drug–drug interactions. Although a brief overview of dosage forms and starting, maintenance and maximum doses is given here, readers are advised to consult the summary of product characteristics (SmPC) for each agent (see References, page 99).

Brivaracetam[1]

Indications. Adjunctive therapy for focal-onset seizures, including focal to bilateral tonic–clonic seizures.

Mechanism of action. Binds to SV2A. The exact role of this protein has yet to be elucidated, but it has been shown to modulate the exocytosis of neurotransmitters.

Dose and administration. Tablets (10 mg, 25 mg, 50 mg, 75 mg, 100 mg). Starting dose: 50 mg/day in two divided doses. Maintenance dose: 50 mg bd. Maximum dose: 100 mg bd.

Contraindications. Rare hereditary galactose intolerance, total lactase deficiency or glucose-galactose malabsorption.

Side effects. Dizziness, tiredness, irritability, anxiety, depression, insomnia, influenza, cough, upper respiratory tract infection and gastrointestinal disturbances. Rare: serious hypersensitivity reactions.

Significant interactions. CBZ, PHT, PB and St John's wort (powerful enzyme inducers) decrease BRV concentrations: dose adjustments are not necessary but use caution with these products. Levels of CBZ metabolite carbamazepine-10,11-epoxide increase substantially: dose adjustment is not necessary but be aware of possible neurotoxic dose-related side effects. Rifampicin reduces BRV concentrations by 45%: dose adjustment of BRV may be required. BRV may increase plasma concentrations of medicinal products transported by organic anion transporter 3 (for example, methotrexate, indomethacin, ciprofloxacin): dose adjustment may be required. BRV approximately doubles the effects of alcohol on psychomotor function, attention and memory: advise patients not to drink much alcohol when taking BRV.

Tips to aid adherence. As with most ASM, slow titration rates reduce the potential for side effects. BRV can be rapidly titrated in urgent clinical situations, but a more conservative approach is warranted in most patients. BRV is better tolerated than LEV (the only other ASM with a similar mode of action) in terms of psychiatric effects. If the patient experiences irritability but the drug otherwise shows promise, then consider adding pyridoxine (vitamin B6), 50–200 mg/day, to try to alleviate these effects. Studies with LEV, while methodologically limited, have shown promise[2] and it is reasonable to extrapolate this benefit to BRV.

Other considerations. BRV is often used to replace LEV when the latter shows promising seizure control but is not well tolerated, particularly if the patient experiences psychiatric side effects. It is acceptable to cross-titrate the drugs, but it is also possible to undertake an overnight switch using a conversion ratio of 10:1 to 15:1.

Cannabidiol

Indications. Adjunctive treatment for seizures associated with LGS or DS for patients 2 years of age and older. Some countries mandate concomitant use of CLB for this indication. Adjunctive therapy for seizures associated with tuberous sclerosis complex (TSC) for patients 2 years of age and older.[3]

Mechanism of action. Precise mechanism of action is unknown. Cannabidiol does not interact with cannabinoid receptors. It reduces neuronal hyperexcitability through modulation of intracellular calcium via G protein-coupled receptor 55 and transient receptor potential vanilloid 1 channels. It also modulates adenosine-mediated signaling through inhibition of adenosine cellular uptake via the equilibrative nucleoside transporter 1.

Dose and administration. Oral solution (100 mg/mL). Starting dose: 5 mg/kg/day in two divided doses. Further increments, not faster than weekly, of 5 mg/kg/day. Maximum dose: 20 mg/kg/day (LGS and DS) or 25 mg/kg/day (TSC).

Contraindications. Hepatocellular injury. Avoid in patients with transaminase elevations greater than three times the upper limit of normal (ULN) and bilirubin greater than two times the ULN. Hypersensitivity to the active substance or to any of the excipients.

Side effects. Most common: diarrhea and vomiting, decreased appetite, somnolence, pyrexia and fatigue. Dosing around food is important (see below). Others include hypersensitivity rashes (may require drug discontinuation if serious), weight reduction, neurotoxic effects such as tiredness, increased liver enzymes, irritability and urinary tract infections.

Significant interactions. Rifampicin may reduce plasma concentrations of cannabidiol by 30–60%. CLB substantially increases the active substances of cannabidiol, enhancing the therapeutic effects but also increasing the risk of neurotoxicity, necessitating CLB dose adjustment. VPA significantly increases the risk of elevated transaminase levels, diarrhea and decreased appetite: dose adjustment of cannabidiol and/or VPA, and in some cases discontinuation, may be required. Theoretical risks of interaction with stiripentol (STP), LTG and PHT: monitor carefully. CBZ, enzalutamide, mitotane and St John's wort may reduce cannabidiol levels significantly: dose adjustment may be required. Drugs affecting the substrates CYP1A2, CYP2B6, CYP2C8, CYP2C9, CYP2C19, UGT1A9 and UGT2B7 (for example, morphine, lorazepam, warfarin and caffeine) may cause clinically significant interactions, though few have been studied: monitor carefully.

Tips to aid adherence. Administer cannabidiol consistently with or without food, and preferably similar types of food each time (for example, if taken with cereal at breakfast, the patient should take it with cereal each time, not a cooked breakfast or toast). Administering cannabidiol with food may increase its bioavailability (and therefore its therapeutic effect) and reduce the incidence of diarrhea, which can be severe. Gastrointestinal disturbances are more common with concomitant administration of VPA. Many patients will be on dual therapy with VPA: careful dose adjustments may be necessary to obtain optimal effects with minimal adverse reactions.

Carbamazepine
Indications. Focal-onset seizures, focal to bilateral tonic–clonic seizures and GTCS. Also, trigeminal neuralgia, prophylaxis of bipolar

disorder unresponsive to lithium. Adjunctive therapy for acute alcohol withdrawal and diabetic neuropathy.[4]

Mechanism of action. CBZ prevents high-frequency repetitive firing of action potentials in depolarized neurons by blocking voltage-dependent sodium channels.

Dose and administration. Sustained- and immediate-release tablets (100 mg. 200 mg, 400 mg), oral suspension and suppositories (short-term use only). Starting dose: 100–200 mg od. Increase by 100–200 mg every 2 weeks. Maintenance dose: 800 mg–1.2 g/day. Maximum dose: 2 g/day. Give sustained-release formulations twice daily. Give immediate-release formulations three times daily.

Contraindications. Acute porphyria, atrioventricular (AV) conduction abnormalities (unless paced) and a history of bone marrow depression.

Side effects. Allergy rash (severe in some cases), including erythema multiforme and Stevens–Johnson syndrome. Test patients of Han Chinese and Thai descent for HLA-B*15:02 to minimize their risk of developing Stevens–Johnson syndrome; avoid CBZ in individuals with positive results. Similar testing for the allele HLA-A*31:01 in patients of European and Japanese descent has been suggested.

Common: mild hyponatremia is usually asymptomatic but can cause confusion, peripheral edema and deterioration in seizure control at sodium levels below 120 mmol/L, requiring dose reduction or drug withdrawal. Reversible mild leukopenia within first few months of treatment: do not discontinue CBZ unless there is evidence of infection or if white blood cell count falls well below 2000×10^9/L. Mild, transient or severe thrombocytopenia: withdraw CBZ if severe. Fluid retention in elderly patients or those with cardiac failure at high concentrations.

Dose-limiting neurotoxic side effects: tiredness, diplopia, headache, dizziness, nausea and vomiting (may occur in the early stages of treatment). Rare: potentially fatal blood dyscrasias and toxic hepatitis.

Significant interactions. Cenobamate (CEN), FBM, fosphenytoin, OXC, PB, PHT, PRM, possibly CZP and herbal remedies such as St John's wort reduce CBZ plasma levels, potentially requiring dose adjustments. VGB increases CBZ plasma concentrations. PRM and VPA increase plasma levels of the CBZ metabolite carbamazepine-10,11-epoxide, but CBZ levels remain stable; consider this if clinical neurotoxicity occurs. CBZ induces metabolism of CLB, CZP, ESM, LTG, ESL, OXC, PRM, TGB, TPM, VPA and ZNS, potentially requiring an increase in dose. Pharmacodynamic interactions can also be important with CBZ, particularly with LEV where symptoms of CBZ toxicity may present.

Consider the OCP ineffective when used concomitantly with CBZ. The progesterone contraceptive implant is similarly affected. Significant interactions with some antimicrobials: erythromycin can reduce carbamazepine-10,11-epoxide levels by 40–60%, compromising seizure control in someone who, by definition, is already unwell.

Interactions with antidepressants and antipsychotics (fluoxetine, fluvoxamine, paroxetine, trazodone and olanzapine): monitor for neurotoxicity or worsening seizure control.

Tips to aid adherence. Autoinduction during initial treatment will result in artificially high levels of CBZ. Warn patients about transient neurotoxic effects; slow titration regimens may help. Sustained-release formulations are preferable, both for improved tolerability and twice-daily rather than three-times-daily administration. Be aware of pharmacodynamic as well as pharmacokinetic interactions, particularly when co-administering with LEV, where it may be necessary to lower the dose of CBZ to avoid neurotoxicity.

Cenobamate

Indications. Focal-onset seizures, including focal to bilateral tonic–clonic seizures.[5]

Mechanism of action. While the precise mechanism of action has yet to be fully elucidated, CEN is a positive allosteric modulator of subtypes of the $GABA_A$ ion channel that does not bind to the benzodiazepine binding site. CEN has also been shown to reduce repetitive neuronal firing by enhancing the inactivation of sodium channels and by inhibiting the persistent component of the sodium current.

Dose and administration. Tablets (12.5 mg, 25 mg, 50 mg, 100 mg, 150 mg, 200 mg). Starting dose: 12.5 mg od for 2 weeks, followed by 25 mg od for 2 weeks, followed by 50 mg od for 2 weeks, then further increments of 50 mg every 2 weeks. Maintenance dose: 200 mg od. Further increments of 50 mg every 2 weeks according to therapeutic response. Maximum dose: 400 mg od.

Contraindications. Familial short QT syndrome.

Side effects. Common: rash. Other: confusion, irritability, tiredness, unsteadiness, nystagmus, gastrointestinal problems and abnormal hepatic function. Rare: severe allergic reaction (DRESS/multiorgan hypersensitivity) associated with faster titration rates, hence the guidance above.

Significant interactions. Increases levels of CLB, PHT and PB: monitor and reduce doses as needed. Decreases concentrations of LTG and CBZ. May need to increase dose of CEN if co-administered with LTG. May significantly reduce the efficacy of oral contraceptives, rendering them ineffective. Possible pharmacodynamic interaction with other CNS depressants, such as barbiturates, alcohol and benzodiazepines, leading to neurotoxicity.

Tips to aid adherence. Emerging experience suggests that slower titration may be advisable to reduce neurotoxic effects, particularly when the patient is taking high-dose polypharmacy.

Clobazam

Indications. Adjunctive treatment in epilepsy and short-term treatment for anxiety.[6]

Mechanism of action. GABA agonist.

Dose and administration. Tablets (10 mg), oral suspension (1 mg/mL, 2 mg/mL, 5 mg/5 mL and 10 mg/5 mL). Starting dose: 10 mg, preferably at night for 1–2 weeks. Increase to 20 mg at night or 10 mg bd, in 10–60 mg dose range depending on efficacy and tolerability.

Twice-daily dosing for doses exceeding 30 mg daily. Maximum dose (in elderly patients): 20 mg/day.

Contraindications. Acute porphyrias, alcohol or drug abuse and severe respiratory depression.

Side effects. Most common: depression, irritability and tiredness. Other: deterioration in behavior and mood disturbance, particularly in patients with ID.

Significant interactions. Low risk of interaction with enzyme-inducing ASM. Increased risk of CNS depression when administered with other drugs with similar CNS side effects, including alcohol, which may affect patient's ability to perform skilled tasks. If awareness is impaired, advise patients not to drive (if eligible to drive) or operate machinery.

Tips to aid adherence. Advise patients to take the higher dose at night if sedation occurs.

Other considerations. Short-term administration (for example, 10–20 mg/day for up to a month or longer, depending on the individual's circumstances) can be an effective strategy in women with catamenial epilepsy who experience cluster seizures (see Chapter 8) and for other patients as 'cover' for holidays or stressful events, such as weddings and surgery. A single dose of 10–30 mg can have a useful prophylactic action if taken immediately after the first event in patients who regularly suffer clusters of focal impaired-awareness and bilateral tonic–clonic seizures.

Clonazepam

Indications. All forms of epilepsy, particularly myoclonic seizures. Also, panic disorders resistant to antidepressants and sleep parasomnias.[7]

Mechanism of action. GABA agonist.

Dose and administration. Tablets (0.5 mg, 2 mg), oral solution (500 mg/5 mL). Starting dose: 0.5–1 mg/night for 4 nights. Increase to 4–8 mg/week, usually taken at night in three or four divided doses.

Contraindications. Acute porphyrias, alcohol or drug abuse and severe respiratory depression.

Side effects. Most common: sedation, ataxia and behavioral changes (for example, depression).

Significant interactions. Low risk of interaction with enzyme-inducing ASM. Increases the risk of CNS depression when administered with other drugs with similar CNS side effects. This may affect the patient's ability to perform skilled tasks. If awareness is impaired, advise the patient not to drive (if eligible to drive) or operate machinery. The effects of alcohol may also be increased and even be felt the next day.

Tips to aid adherence. Advise patients to take CZP at night if sedation occurs.

Eslicarbazepine acetate
Indications for use. Monotherapy and adjunctive treatment for focal-onset seizures with or without bilateral tonic–clonic seizures.[8]

Mechanism of action. Voltage-gated sodium-channel blocker.

Dose and administration. Tablets (200 mg, 800 mg), oral solution (50 mg/mL). Starting dose: 400 mg od for 1–2 weeks. Increase to 800 mg od according to response. Maintenance dose: 800–1200 mg od.

Contraindications. Second- or third-degree AV block.

Side effects. Most common: dizziness, somnolence, headache, abnormal coordination, disturbed attention, tremor, diplopia, blurred vision, vertigo, nausea, vomiting and diarrhea. Patients taking CBZ and ESL may experience diplopia, abnormal coordination and dizziness more often than with other combinations. Hyponatremia occurs less frequently with ESL than with CBZ and much less frequently than with OXC. Risk of Stevens–Johnson syndrome rash.

Significant interactions. Co-administration with PHT reduces ESL concentrations with increased PHT levels: may need PHT dose adjustment. Interacts with the combined OCP and can cause pill failure.

Tips to aid adherence. When administering with CBZ, consider reducing the CBZ dose so that the patient may better tolerate ESL. Give the daily dose at night to avoid neurotoxic effects associated with peak plasma concentrations.

Other considerations. Use cautiously in patients at risk of hyponatremia and with other drugs that can cause a prolonged PR interval.

Ethosuximide

Indications. Monotherapy for absence and myoclonic seizures, and adjunctive treatment for atypical absence seizures.[9]

Mechanism of action. Reduces T-type calcium currents in thalamic neurons.

Dose and administration. Capsules (250 mg), oral solution (250 mg/5 mL). Starting dose: 250 mg bd for 1 week. Increase by 250 mg/day every week according to response. Maintenance dose: 1–2 g daily in divided doses.

Contraindications. Acute porphyrias.

Side effects. Most common: hiccups, nausea, vomiting, abdominal pain and anorexia. Other: headache, dizziness, drowsiness and unsteadiness. Rare: blood disorders. Advise patients who experience fever, unexplained bruising and bleeding or mouth ulcers to seek medical attention. Risk of Stevens-Johnson syndrome rash.

Significant interactions. Levels are often (but not always) increased by VPA and reduced by CBZ, PHT, PRM and PB, as well as LTG: dose adjustment and/or plasma level monitoring may be required. Levels are also increased by isoniazide.

Other considerations. Generally used for the control of absences. It does not usually control GTCS in adults, in which case additional treatment with a broad-spectrum ASM is required. VPA, unless contraindicated, is normally the first choice. Do not use ESM in focal epilepsy.

Felbamate

Indications. Adjunctive therapy and monotherapy for focal seizures, including focal to bilateral tonic–clonic seizures. Also, adjunctive treatment for seizures associated with LGS.[10]

Mechanism of action. FBM potentiates GABA activity and blocks voltage-dependent sodium channels as well as the ion channel at the N-methyl-D-aspartate (NMDA) excitatory amino acid receptor.

Dose and administration. Tablets (400 mg, 600 mg), oral solution (600 mg/5 mL). Initiate slowly and titrate over several weeks to minimize side effects. Doses of 1800–4800 mg/day are usually necessary for optimal seizure control.

Contraindications. Blood dyscrasia and hepatic dysfunction.

Side effects. Warning: FBM is not available in many countries because of the risk of aplastic anemia and hepatotoxicity. It is now largely restricted to patients with LGS for whom the benefits of treatment outweigh the risks. Other: insomnia, headache, nausea, anorexia, somnolence, vomiting, weight loss and dizziness.

Significant interactions. Increases serum concentrations of PHT, VPA, PB and carbamazepine-10, 11-epoxide. Lowers the concentration of CBZ. PHT, PB and CBZ lower FBM levels, while VPA increases FBM levels. Dose adjustment of the concomitant ASM is usually necessary when FBM is introduced. Renders the OCP ineffective. Significant interaction with other drugs metabolized by the CYP450 system.

Gabapentin

Indications. Monotherapy and adjunctive treatment for focal-onset seizures with or without bilateral tonic–clonic seizures. Also, treatment of peripheral neuropathic pain.[11]

Mechanism of action. GBP binds the $\alpha_2\delta$ subunit of the neuronal voltage-gated calcium channels, inhibiting calcium flow and neurotransmitter release from presynaptic neurons.

Dose and administration. Tablets (600 mg, 800 mg), capsules (100 mg, 300 mg, 400 mg), oral solution (50 mg/mL). Starting dose: 300–400 mg od for 1–3 days. Increase to 300–400 mg bd for 1–3 days, then increase by 300–400 mg/day at 1–2-week intervals according to response. Maintenance dose: 0.9–3.6 g/day in three divided doses.

Side effects. Most common: drowsiness, ataxia, dizziness and nystagmus. Other: weight gain (at higher doses), flatulence and diarrhea. Can worsen absence and myoclonic jerks in generalized epilepsies (in preclinical studies of patients with focal-onset epilepsy, up to 20% also noticed worsening seizure control).[12] No idiosyncratic reactions or effects on bone marrow or hepatic function.

Significant interactions. Slows FBM clearance. Rare risk of severe respiratory depression when used in combination with opioid medicines and other CNS depressants, particularly in elderly patients. Advise patients of interaction between GBP and alcohol and the risk of CNS depression. Antacids containing aluminum and magnesium reduce GBP bioavailability by up to 24%: take GBP at least 2 hours after antacid administration.

Tips to aid adherence. 1–2 weekly titration rates, rather than 1–3 days, along with lower initial doses.

Other considerations. Take care when using GBP in elderly patients and those with severe respiratory depression, a history of drug and alcohol abuse, and congestive cardiac failure. In the UK, GBP is classified as a Class C controlled substance and a Schedule 3 drug because of concerns about abuse. In the USA, GBP is not a federally controlled substance but it is a Schedule V controlled drug in some states. Check for a history of drug abuse before prescribing and observe for signs of abuse and dependence. Use high doses of the oral solution with caution in patients with diabetes mellitus or low bodyweight, as levels of propylene glycol, acesulfame K and saccharin sodium are high.

Lacosamide

Indications. Monotherapy and adjunctive treatment for focal-onset seizures with or without bilateral tonic–clonic seizures.[13]

Mechanism of action. LCM enhances the slow inactivation of voltage-gated sodium channels.

Dose and administration. Tablets (50 mg, 100 mg, 150 mg, 200 mg), oral solution (10 mg/mL), solution for infusion (200 mg/20 mL). Starting dose: 50 mg bd for 2 weeks. Increase by 50 mg/day at 2-week intervals according to response. Maintenance dose: 200–400 mg in divided doses.

Contraindications. Second- or third-degree AV block. Ensure patients have ECG before treatment and use caution when taking other medicinal products associated with PR prolongation.

Side effects. Most common: dizziness, headache, diplopia, nausea, vomiting, fatigue, blurred vision, poor coordination, somnolence, tremor and nystagmus.

Significant interactions. PHT, PB and CBZ may reduce LCM concentrations.

Tips to aid adherence. Titrate slowly, starting at 50 mg at night for 2 weeks, increasing to 50 mg bd.

Other considerations. Use caution in elderly patients because of the risk of PR-interval prolongation and severe cardiac disease.

Lamotrigine

Indications. Adjunctive treatment and monotherapy for focal-onset seizures with or without bilateral tonic–clonic seizures, GTCS and seizures associated with LGS.[14]

Mechanism of action. LTG selectively blocks the slow inactivated state of the sodium channel, thereby preventing the release of excitatory amino acid neurotransmitters, particularly glutamate and aspartate.

Dose and administration. Tablets (25 mg, 50 mg, 100 mg, 200 mg), dispersible tablets (2 mg, 5 mg, 25 mg, 100 mg). Starting dose: 25 mg od for 2 weeks. Increase to 50 mg od for 2 weeks, and then increase by 50 mg every 2 weeks according to response. Maintenance dose: 200–500 mg/day in divided doses.

In adjunctive treatment with VPA, give an initial dose of 25 mg od on alternate days for 2 weeks, then increase to 25 mg od for 2 weeks, and then by 50 mg every 2 weeks. Maintenance dose: 100–200 mg/day in divided doses.

Side effects. Most common: headache, nausea, insomnia, vomiting, dizziness, diplopia, ataxia and tremor. Seldom causes sedation. Rash complicates initial management in about 3% of patients taking LTG monotherapy and 8% of those already established on VPA. It is usually maculopapular and, in mild cases, may subside spontaneously without drug withdrawal. A few patients have an accompanying systemic illness with malaise, fever, arthralgia, myalgia, lymphadenopathy and eosinophilia. Cases of bullous erythema multiforme, Stevens–Johnson syndrome and toxic epidermal necrolysis have been reported.

Significant interactions. When used as monotherapy, the half-life of LTG is approximately 24 hours. When given to patients already being treated with CBZ, PHT or PB, the half-life falls to about 15 hours. VPA inhibits glucuronidation of LTG, prolonging its half-life to around 60 hours. Withdrawal of enzyme-inducing ASM therefore causes a rise in the circulating concentrations of LTG, while discontinuing VPA produces a fall. Neurotoxicity (headache, dizziness, nausea, diplopia, ataxia) is common when LTG is introduced in patients established on high-dose CBZ or OXC: stagger doses of CBZ or OXC and LTG by 2–3 hours instead of administering them simultaneously. A pharmacodynamic interaction may also explain the marked tremor seen in some patients taking VPA and LTG in combination.

In combination with the OCP, LTG levels can fall by over 50%. Dose adjustment may be required. In practice, this can be problematic because of the 'pill-free week' when LTG concentrations would be significantly higher, possibly resulting in neurotoxicity. LTG also reduces progesterone levels by about 20%, but this is not thought to result in ovulation.

Rifampicin, lopinavir, ritonavir and atanzavir can reduce plasma concentrations of LTG: dose adjustment may be required.

Tips to aid adherence. Advise patients who have vivid dreams/sleep disturbance to take nighttime dose earlier. Use slower titration rates when LTG is added to VPA: smaller doses are available in dispersible form.

Other considerations. Serum concentrations of LTG fall during pregnancy: monitor concentrations and adjust dose accordingly.

Levetiracetam

Indications. Monotherapy and adjunctive treatment for focal-onset seizures with or without bilateral tonic–clonic seizures. Also, adjunctive treatment for myoclonic, GTCS and SE (see Chapter 7).[15]

Mechanism of action. SV2A ligand.

Dose and administration. Tablets (250 mg, 500 mg, 750 mg, 1000 mg), granules (250 mg, 500 mg, 1000 mg), oral solution (100 mg/mL), solution for infusion (500 mg/5 mL). Starting dose: 250 mg od for 1–2 weeks, then 250 mg bd. Increase by 250 mg bd every 2 weeks according to response. Maintenance dose: 1–3 g/day in divided doses.

Side effects. Most common: tiredness, anxiety, agitation, aggression, emotional lability, hostility, psychosis and depression, particularly in patients with a history of ID and dementia. Other: headache, weight change and gastrointestinal discomfort. Rare: idiosyncratic skin rash.

Significant interactions. Decreases clearance of methotrexate: monitor LEV and methotrexate concentrations.

Tips to aid adherence. Reduce the risk of behavioral side effects by slower titration and limiting the dose. In addition, pyridoxine (vitamin B6), 50–200 mg/day helps to alleviate mood-related side effects, though many of the studies in this area are not robust.[2]

Other considerations. As levetiracetam can worsen psychiatric symptoms, it should be used with caution in patients with anxiety, depression, suicidal ideation and dementia.

Midazolam

Indications. SE (see Chapter 7).[16]

Mechanism of action. GABA agonist.

Dose and administration. Oromucosal solution, solution for injection and solution for infusion (10 mg). Starting dose: 10 mg. If no response after 10 minutes, administer another 10 mg.

Contraindications. CNS and respiratory depression in patients whose airway is compromised.

Side effects. Respiratory depression, hypotension and sedation.

Significant interactions. Low risk of interaction with enzyme-inducing ASM. Increases the risk of CNS depression when administered with other drugs with similar CNS side effects, which may affect the patient's ability to perform skilled tasks.

Other considerations. See Chapter 7 on management of seizures in a community setting and the training requirements for family members and carers.

Oxcarbazepine

Indications. Monotherapy and adjunctive treatment of focal-onset seizures with or without bilateral tonic–clonic seizures.[17]

Mechanism of action. Sodium channel blocker. OXC also modulates calcium and potassium currents.

Dose and administration. Tablets (150 mg, 300 mg, 600 mg), oral suspension (60 mg/mL). Starting dose: 150 mg bd. Increase by 300–600 mg/day every 2 weeks according to response. Maintenance dose: 0.6–2.4 g/day in divided doses.

Contraindications. Acute porphyrias.

Side effects. Most common: CNS side effects, including drowsiness, dizziness, headache, diplopia, nausea, vomiting and ataxia. Other: depression, mood changes, cognitive impairment, hyponatremia and rash (less frequently than with CBZ). Rare: Stevens–Johnson syndrome and blood disorders.

Significant interactions. Interactions are similar to CBZ, but OXC is a less potent enzyme inducer so the interactions, and therefore the implications for treatment, are less marked. Reduces the effect of the OCP.

Tips to aid adherence. If a twice daily dose cannot be tolerated, OXC can be taken three times a day.

Other considerations. Regularly test plasma sodium concentration in patients at risk of hyponatremia. Monitor bodyweight in patients with heart failure.

Perampanel

Indications. Adjunctive treatment for focal-onset seizures with or without bilateral tonic–clonic seizures and for GTCS.[18]

Mechanism of action. A unique, highly selective, non-competitive antagonist of the ionotropic α-amino-3-hydroxy-5-methyl-4-isoxazolepropionic acid (AMPA) glutamate receptor on postsynaptic neurons. Activation of AMPA receptors by glutamate is thought to be responsible for most fast excitatory synaptic transmission in the brain. Precise mechanism of action is not fully known.

Dose and administration. Tablets (2 mg, 4 mg, 6 mg, 8 mg, 10 mg, 12 mg), oral suspension (0.5 mg/mL). Starting dose: 2 mg od at night.

Increase by 2 mg/day at 2-week intervals if tolerated and according to response to 6 mg at night. Maximum dose: 6–12 mg every night.

Contraindications. None, but avoid in patients with severe hepatic and renal impairment.

Side effects. Dizziness, somnolence, nausea, diplopia, ataxia, vertigo, headache, decreased and increased appetite, fatigue, gait disturbance and falls. Psychiatric disorders such as aggression, anger, anxiety and confusion are not uncommon.

Significant interactions. PHT, CBZ and OXC decrease levels: adjust dose as necessary. In particular, CBZ increases PER clearance up to threefold. PER does not seem to affect the metabolism of other ASM. At high doses PER decreases levanorgestrol but not ethinylestradiol exposure. Possibility of decreased efficacy of progesterone-containing oral contraceptives in women established on PER, 12 mg/day.

Tips to aid adherence. Much slower titration rates than those in the SmPC are vital. The authors' experience suggests starting at 2 mg od, increasing to 4 mg od after 4 weeks. Continue titration no faster than 4 mg every 4 weeks until seizure control is established. For some people, particularly those with ID, try even slower regimens. Given the drug's half-life of around 120 hours, it is feasible to start the drug at 2 mg once every other day or even once every 3 days to alleviate side effects. It is very important to give PER at bedtime to avoid the neurotoxicity associated with peak plasma concentrations.

Other considerations. PER has by far the longest half-life of any ASM. This may make it particularly helpful for people who find it difficult to remember to take medication.

Phenobarbital
Indications. All forms of epilepsy except for absence seizures. Also, SE (see Chapter 7).[19]

Mechanism of action. GABA agonist.

Dose and administration. Tablets (15 mg, 30 mg or 60 mg), oral solution (15 mg/5 mL), solution for injection (30 mg/1 mL). Maintenance dose: 60–180 mg od, given as tablets

Contraindications. Acute porphyrias. Avoid use in elderly patients and those with a history of drug and alcohol abuse or respiratory depression, as it can cause CNS-depressant effects.

Side effects. Common: sedation and behavioral problems, such as anxiety, depression and agitation. Other: cognitive impairment, memory loss, risk of allergic rash, osteoporosis, folate deficiency and Dupuytren's contracture.

Significant interactions. OXC, PHT and VPA increase PB plasma concentrations. Monitor patients being treated concomitantly with VPA for signs of hyperammonemia (half of reported cases are asymptomatic and do not necessarily result in clinical encephalopathy). VGB possibly decreases PB plasma concentrations. PB is a powerful inducer of hepatic metabolism, accelerating the clearance of many other lipid-soluble drugs. It renders the OCP ineffective.

Tips to aid adherence. Patients who cannot tolerate one daily dose may take PB in two or three divided doses.

Other considerations. PB is no longer considered first-line treatment because of its significant side effects and many clinically relevant interactions. However, advise people who have been taking PB for many years without problems to remain on it rather than to switch to a newer ASM. It still has a role in drug-resistant epilepsy and is cheap and therefore readily available in developing economies.

Phenytoin
Indications. Focal-onset seizures with or without bilateral tonic–clonic seizures. It can also be given during and after neurosurgery or severe head injury to prevent and treat seizures. Also, SE (see Chapter 7).[20]

Mechanism of action. Sodium channel blocker.

Dose and administration. Tablets (100 mg), chewable tablets (50 mg), capsules (25 mg, 50 mg, 100 mg, 300 mg), oral suspension (30 mg/5 mL), solution for injection (250 mg/5 mL). Starting dose: 150–300 mg od. Increase according to therapeutic response. Maintenance dose: 200–500 mg (alternatively 3–4 mg/kg/day) with or after food.

Contraindications. Acute porphyrias, sinus bradycardia, second- and third-degree heart block and Adams–Stokes syndrome.

Side effects. Neurotoxic symptoms (ataxia, nystagmus, dysarthria, asterixis, somnolence) typically present 8–12 hours after an oral dose. Chronic dysmorphic effects (gingival hyperplasia, hirsutism, acne, facial coarsening) occur after months of treatment. Uncommon long-term problems (folate deficiency, osteopenia, peripheral neuropathy, cerebellar atrophy) take years to develop. Other: Stevens–Johnson syndrome rash. Rare: hepatitis, bone marrow suppression, lymphadenopathy and a lupus-like syndrome

Significant interactions. PHT reduces serum concentrations of CBZ, VPA, LTG, PER and TPM. PHT is tightly bound to circulating albumin and may be displaced by other drugs; some of these, such as VPA, also inhibit the metabolism of PHT. PHT's induction of hepatic enzymes may also reduce the effectiveness of other lipid-soluble drugs, including oral contraceptives and anticoagulants.

Tips to aid adherence. Treat patients with erratic adherence twice daily to lessen the effect of a missed dose.

Other considerations. PHT has non-linear pharmacokinetics, so small dose adjustments can have large effects on plasma concentrations. Assess plasma levels after dose changes, treatment with concomitant drugs that interact and routinely every 12 months. Let plasma levels guide dosage.

Pregabalin
Indications. Adjunctive treatment for focal-onset seizures with or without bilateral tonic–clonic seizures.[21]

Mechanism of action. PGB has an amino acid configuration and is structurally related to GABA. Like GBP, it binds with high affinity to the $\alpha_2\delta$ subunit of neuronal voltage-gated calcium channels.

Dose and administration. Tablets and capsules (25 mg, 50 mg, 75 mg, 100 mg, 150 mg, 200 mg, 225 mg, 300 mg), oral solution (20 mg/mL). Starting dose: 25 mg bd. Increase by 50 mg/day every 1–2 weeks according to response to 300 mg/day in two or three divided doses. Maximum dose: 600 mg/day in two or three divided doses.

Side effects. Most common: dizziness, somnolence, asthenia, headache and ataxia. Other: weight gain (particularly at high doses), gastrointestinal disorders, mood changes and nausea.

Significant interactions. Use caution when administering PGB with other ASM that may have CNS-depressant effects, including CBZ, CZP, CEN and lorazepam. Risk of CNS and respiratory depression with other drugs that cause CNS depression, such as opioids.

Tips to aid adherence. Advise patients to take PGB in two or three divided doses and to avoid alcohol.

Other considerations. Be careful when using PGB in patients with severe respiratory depression, elderly patients, and those with a history of drug and alcohol abuse or congestive cardiac failure. In the UK, PGB is classified as a Class C controlled substance and a Schedule 3 drug because of concerns about abuse. In the USA it is a Schedule V controlled drug. Check for a history of drug abuse before prescribing and observe for signs of misuse and dependence. Advise patients about the interaction between PGB and alcohol and its risk of causing CNS depression.

Primidone
Indications for use. All forms of epilepsy.[22]

Mechanism of action is not fully understood. However, it is metabolized in the liver to PB and another active substance, phenylethylmalonamide.

Dose and administration. Tablets (50 mg, 250 mg), oral suspension (125 mg/5 mL). Starting dose: 125 mg at night. Increase by 125 mg every 3–5 days as tolerated and according to therapeutic response. Maintenance dose: 500–1500 mg/day in two or three divided doses.

Contraindications. Acute porphyrias. Use with caution in elderly patients and patients with a history of drug and alcohol abuse, as PRM can have CNS-depressant effects.

Side effects. Most common: ataxia, dizziness, nausea and visual impairment.

Significant interactions. PRM may decrease plasma concentrations of CBZ, FBM, LTG, OXC, PER, PHT (with the additional risk of increased PB concentrations and possible toxicity, as well as possible toxicity with PHT on stopping PRM), STP, TGB, VPA and ZNS. OXC may decrease PRM plasma levels. Reduces the effect of the OCP. Isoniazid and nicotinamide cause very high levels of PRM, with neurotoxic side effects. Expect similar interactions as seen with PB, because PRM is metabolized to PB.

Tips to aid adherence. Be mindful of drug interactions, particularly if PHT or CBZ are added to existing PRM therapy, which can raise therapeutic levels to toxic levels. Use much lower titration regimens in clinical practice than those published in formularies, as acute adverse reactions can occur in the early stages of treatment.

Other considerations. Rather like PB, PRM is no longer considered a first-line ASM. However, if a patient has been stable on PRM for many years, it may be better to maintain treatment than switch to a newer ASM. The half-life of PRM is short (3.3–11 hours), and three-times-daily dosing may be appropriate, though in clinical practice a twice-daily regimen is usually preferred.

Rufinamide

Indications. Adjunctive treatment for seizures associated with LGS.[23]

Mechanism of action. RFN is a triazole derivative that reduces the recovery capacity of neuronal sodium channels after inactivation, thereby limiting action potential firing. Other unknown mechanisms of action are also likely given the drug's broad-spectrum antiepileptic properties.

Dose and administration. Tablets (100 mg, 200 mg, 400 mg), oral suspension (40 mg/mL). Starting dose, in adjunctive treatment without VPA: 200 mg bd. Increased by 200–400 mg/day in divided doses according to therapeutic response. Maintenance dose: 1.2 g bd. Starting dose in adjunctive treatment with VPA: 200 mg bd. Increase by 200–400 mg/day in divided doses according to therapeutic response. Maintenance dose: 800 mg bd.

Contraindications. Shortened QTc interval.

Side effects. Common: headache, dizziness, fatigue and somnolence. Other: nausea, vomiting, anxiety, insomnia and weight gain. Rare: hypersensitivity reactions with fever, rash and lymphadenopathy.

Significant interactions. VPA can significantly increase RFN plasma levels. RFN may reduce the clearance, and hence increase the circulating concentrations, of PHT. Induces the metabolism of ethinylestradiol and norethisterone in the combined OCP.

Tips to aid adherence. Tablets can be crushed and swallowed with water.

Other considerations. RFN has orphan drug status for LGS because it is particularly effective against tonic and atonic seizures. These can cause devastating falls and injuries, so while another ASM may be required, RFN can be an effective adjunct.

Sodium valproate

Indications. All forms of epilepsy, particularly GGE. Also, SE (see Chapter 7).[24]

Mechanism of action. VPA limits sustained repetitive firing via a use- and voltage-dependent effect on sodium and calcium channels. It also facilitates the effects of GABA and NMDA receptor antagonism.

Dose and administration. Tablets and modified-release tablets (200 mg, 300 mg, 500 mg), 200 mg, gastroresistant tablets (500 mg), modified-release capsules (150 mg, 300 mg), modified-release granules (50 mg, 100 mg, 250 mg, 500 mg, 750 mg, 1000 mg), oral solution (200 mg/5 mL), solution for injection (300 mg/3 mL), powder and solvent solution for injection (400 mg/4 mL). Starting dose: 500–600 mg od or bd for 1 week. Increase by 200–400 mg every 1–2 weeks according to therapeutic response. Maintenance dose: 1–2 g/day. Maximum dose: 2.5 g/day; alternatively, titrate VPA according to the person's weight, 20–30 mg/kg daily.

Contraindications. Acute porphyrias. Ideally, avoid in pregnancy because of significant risk of birth defects and developmental disorders (10% birth defects and 30–40% risk of developmental delay[25]). VPA is the ASM associated with the highest risk of congenital malformation in several epilepsy and pregnancy registries,[26] but do not stop VPA abruptly if a woman becomes pregnant. If a woman who is stable on VPA is planning a pregnancy, ensure she discusses her ongoing use of VPA with an epilepsy specialist.

Side effects. Most common: dose-related tremor, weight gain due to appetite stimulation, abdominal pain, thinning or loss of hair (usually temporary) and menstrual irregularities including amenorrhea. Other: some young women develop polycystic ovary syndrome associated with obesity and hirsutism. Rare: stupor and encephalopathy associated with hyperammonemia, thrombocytopenia (can be severe) and hepatic toxicity (can be severe).

Significant interactions. Inhibits a range of hepatic metabolic processes, including oxidation, conjugation and epoxidation reactions, particularly for PHT, PB, carbamazepine-10,11-epoxide and LTG. VPA and LTG dual therapy is effective but adjust dose of LTG to prevent toxicity. Increases exposure to RFN. Risk of hepatotoxicity with statins such as atorvastatin and simvastatin, antibiotics such as doxycycline, flucloxacillin and oxytetracycline, immunosuppressants such as methotrexate, and analgesics such as acetaminophen (paracetamol). Withdraw VPA immediately if patient experiences hepatic dysfunction with persistent vomiting, abdominal pain, weight loss, jaundice and deterioration in seizure control. Also withdraw immediately if patient develops pancreatitis.

Tips to aid adherence. Introduce slowly in divided doses, especially when adding to LTG. Patients who often forget morning or evening medication when the drug is given in divided doses, can take one dose at night, though the normal half-life range for adults (12–15 hours) would theoretically preclude this. Modified-release preparations (tablets or granules) prolong the half-life slightly and are probably better tolerated than enteric coated preparations and therefore preferred.

Stiripentol

Indications. Adjunctive therapy in combination with VPA and CLB in drug-resistant GTCS and severe myoclonic epilepsy in infancy – Dravet syndrome (DS).[27]

Mechanism of action. Enhances central GABAergic neurotransmission by increasing GABA release, thereby prolonging the inhibitory effect of GABA.

Dose and administration. Capsules (250 mg, 500 mg), powder sachets for an oral suspension. Starting dose: 50 mg/kg/day bd or tid, preferably during meals. Increase as necessary. Maximum dose: 3500 mg/day.

Contraindications. History of psychosis.

Side effects. Most common: drowsiness, slowing of cognitive function, ataxia, diplopia, anorexia, weight loss, nausea, abdominal pain and asymptomatic neutropenia

Significant interactions. Increases the concentration of CBZ, PHT, PRM, diazepam, ESM, TGB and PB: requires careful monitoring and potential dose adjustment. Dose-dependent adverse reactions with statins. Take care when combining with midazolam, trazolam and alprazolam because of increased plasma benzodiazepine levels leading to excessive sedation. A similar effect may be seen with chlorpromazine.

Other considerations. The manufacturer advises against ingesting milk and dairy products, carbonated drinks, fruit juices or caffeine-containing food and drinks at the same time. Capsules and oral powder are not bioequivalent: monitor switching because of the risk of toxicity.

Tiagabine

Indications. Adjunctive treatment for focal-onset seizures with or without bilateral tonic–clonic seizures.[28]

Mechanism of action. TGB selectively inhibits the neuronal and glial reuptake of GABA, thereby enhancing GABA-mediated inhibition.

Dose and administration. Tablets (5 mg, 10 mg, 15 mg). Starting dose: 5–10 mg od or bd for 2 weeks. Increase by 5–10 mg every 2 weeks in two or three divided doses according to therapeutic response. Maintenance dose: 30–45 mg/day with enzyme-inducing ASM; 15–30 mg/day with non-enzyme-inducing ASM.

Contraindications. Acute porphyrias.

Side effects. Most common: dizziness, asthenia, nervousness, tremor, impaired concentration, lethargy and depression. Weakness due to transient loss of tone at high doses. The most common reasons for discontinuation of therapy are confusion, somnolence, ataxia and dizziness. Other: acute psychotic reactions, particularly in patients with a history of psychiatric disease.

Significant interactions. CBZ, PHT and PB decrease exposure to TGB, thereby lowering its plasma concentrations. St John's wort is contraindicated as it significantly reduces levels of TGB, leading to a loss of efficacy.

Tips to aid adherence. Advise patients to take TGB with or just after food to avoid rapid rises in plasma concentration.

Other considerations. TGB may worsen absence, myoclonic, tonic and atonic seizures.

Topiramate

Indications. Monotherapy and adjunctive treatment for focal-onset seizures with or without bilateral tonic–clonic seizures and GTCS. Also, adjunctive treatment for patients with LGS.[29] Also, prophylactic treatment for migraine.

Mechanism of action. TPM is a sulfamate-substituted monosaccharide that has multiple pharmacological actions involving blockade of sodium channels and high-voltage-activated calcium channels, attenuation of kainate-induced responses and enhancement of GABAergic neurotransmission. It also inhibits carbonic anhydrase, an effect that contributes to its side-effect profile.

Dose and administration. Tablets (25 mg, 50 mg, 100 mg, 200 mg), capsules (15 mg, 25 mg, 50 mg), oral suspension (50 mg/5 mL, 100 mg/5 mL). Starting dose: 25–50 mg at night for the first week. Increase by 25–50 mg every 2 weeks in divided doses according to therapeutic response. Maintenance dose: 200–400 mg/day in divided doses.

Contraindications. Acute porphyrias and history of kidney stones (risk of metabolic acidosis and nephrolithiasis).

Side effects. Most common: ataxia, poor concentration, confusion, dysphasia, dizziness, fatigue, paresthesia, somnolence, word-finding difficulties, cognitive slowing, anorexia and weight loss. Other: acute glaucoma, kidney stones (in 1 in 10 men) which can cause severe abdominal pain, constipation and high blood pressure, and acute psychotic reactions, particularly in patients with a history of psychiatric disease.

Significant interactions. Increases the risk of CBZ toxicity. CBZ, PB and PHT decrease TPM concentrations and TPM decreases PHT concentrations. TPM at doses over 200 mg daily decreases the efficacy of estrogen and can lead to contraceptive failure for women taking an OCP. Exercise caution when using TPM concomitantly with carbonic anhydrase inhibitors such as ZNS and acetazolomide because of the possibility of a pharmacodynamic interaction, most concerningly increasing the risk of kidney stones.

Tips to aid adherence. Minimize the risk of neurocognitive side effects by titrating slowly. The contents of a capsule can be sprinkled on soft food and swallowed without chewing to aid adherence.

Vigabatrin

Indications. Adjunctive treatment for focal-onset seizures with or without bilateral tonic–clonic seizures.[30]

Mechanism of action. Inhibits GABA transaminase, the enzyme responsible for the metabolic degradation of GABA.

Dose and administration. Tablets (500 mg), powder for oral solution (500 mg). Starting dose: 500 mg bd for 2 weeks. Increase by 500 mg every 2 weeks according to therapeutic response. Maintenance dose: 2000–3000 mg/day.

Contraindications. Visual field defects affect up to 40% of patients. The onset of visual impairment varies from 1 month to a few years and visual field defects persist and may worsen despite VGB discontinuation. Conduct visual field testing before starting treatment and at 6-monthly intervals.

Side effects. Most common: tiredness, dizziness, headache and weight gain. Other: mood changes (commonly agitation, ill temper, disturbed behavior or depression), and acute psychotic reactions, particularly in patients with a history of psychiatric disease.

Significant interactions. Reduces the concentration of PHT.

Other considerations. Can worsen absences and myoclonic jerks.

Zonisamide

Indications. Monotherapy for focal-onset seizures with or without bilateral tonic–clonic seizures in newly diagnosed epilepsy. Adjunctive treatment for drug-resistant focal-onset seizures with or without bilateral tonic–clonic seizures.[31]

Mechanism of action. Blocks voltage-dependent sodium and T-type calcium channels, and actively inhibits the release of excitatory neurotransmitters.

Dose and administration. Capsules (25 mg, 50 mg, 100 mg), oral suspension (20 mg/mL). Starting dose: 25 mg bd for 2 weeks. Increase to 50 mg bd for 2 weeks, and further increase by 50 mg/day at 2-week intervals. Maintenance dose: 300–500 mg/day in one or two divided doses.

Contraindications. Theoretical hypersensitivity syndrome, such as a risk of rash.

Side effects. Most common: anxiety, mood changes, decreased appetite, weight loss, cognitive impairment, somnolence, gastrointestinal discomfort, dizziness, ataxia and fatigue. Uncommon: behavioral changes and, gallbladder disorders and rarely reported agranulocytosis, angle closure glaucoma and renal failure.

Significant interactions. PHT, CBZ and PB decrease the half-life of ZNS by approximately 50%. LTG increases ZNS concentrations. ZNS can reduce carbamazepine-10,11-epoxide ratio. Use ZNS with caution in adults treated concomitantly with carbonic anhydrase inhibitors such as TPM and acetazolamide, as there are insufficient data to rule out a possible pharmacodynamic interaction. Most worrying is an increased risk of kidney stones.

Tips to aid adherence. Use a slower titration if necessary. ZNS's relatively long half-life (49–69 hours in monotherapy) means that once-daily administration is possible, particularly when a stable dose has been reached.

Other considerations. Patients with renal dysfunction have lower rates of clearance, so discontinue ZNS if renal function deteriorates. Exercise caution in elderly patients with a history of eye disorders and low bodyweight.

 Key points – antiseizure medications

- There are now multiple types of ASM for the management of epilepsies available in different pharmaceutical forms; oral administration is the mainstay of ASM delivery.
- Careful attention must be paid to interactions between ASM and with other drugs; some ASM have large numbers of clinically relevant interactions and it is advisable to consult the appropriate SmPC in these cases.
- In some circumstances it may be appropriate to titrate doses more slowly than recommended in an ASM's SmPC, particularly if the patient has a history of poor tolerability to ASM.
- Some ASM may cause acute psychotic reactions in patients with a history of psychiatric disease.
- VPA should ideally be avoided in pregnancy, in consultation with an epilepsy specialist, because of its association with a significant risk of birth defects and developmental disorders.

References

1. European Medicines Agency. *Summary of product characteristics: brivaracetam.* European Medicines Agency, ?. www.ema.europa.eu/ en/documents/product-information/briviact-epar-product-information_en.pdf, last accessed 7 March 2022.

2. Romoli M, Perucca E, Sen A. Pyridoxine supplementation for levetiracetam-related neuropsychiatric adverse events: a systematic review. *Epilepsy Behav* 2020;103:106861.

3. Electronic Medicines Compendium. *Epidyolex 100 mg/ml oral solution: summary of product characteristics.* Electronic Medicines Compendium, 2022. www.medicines.org.uk/emc/ product/10781/smpc, last accessed 7 March 2022.

4. Electronic Medicines Compendium. *Tegretol 100 mg tablets: summary of product characteristics.* Electronic Medicines Compendium, 2021. www.medicines.org.uk/ emc/product/1040/smpc, last accessed 7 March 2022.

5. Electronic Medicines Compendium. *Ontozry 200 mg film-coated tablets: summary of product characteristics.* Electronic Medicines Compendium, 2021. www.medicines.org.uk/emc/ product/13012/smpc, last accessed 7 March 2022.

6. Electronic Medicines Compendium. *Clobazam Accord 10 mg tablets: summary of product characteristics.* Electronic Medicines Compendium, 2020. www.medicines.org.uk/ emc/product/5029/smpc, last accessed 7 March 2022.

7. Electronic Medicines Compendium. *Clonazepam Rosemont 0.5 mg/5 ml oral solution: summary of product characteristics.* Electronic Medicines Compendium, 2020. www.medicines.org.uk/ emc/product/6021/smpc, last accessed 9 March 2022.

8. Electronic Medicines Compendium. *Zebinix 200 mg tablets: summary of product characteristics.* Electronic Medicines Compendium, 2021. www.medicines.org.uk/ emc/product/4460/smpc, last accessed 7 March 2022.

9. Electronic Medicines Compendium. *Ethosuximide Essential Generics 250 mg capsules: summary of product characteristics.* Electronic Medicines Compendium, 2021. www.medicines.org.uk/emc/ product/12896/smpc, last accessed 9 March 2022.

10. Drugs.com. *Felbamate.* Drugs. com, 2022. www.drugs.com/ pro/felbamate.html, last accessed 8 March 2022.

11. Electronic Medicines Compendium. *Gabapentin 300mg capsules: summary of product characteristics*. Electronic Medicines Compendium, 2022. www.medicines.org.uk/emc/product/4636/smpc, last accessed 8 March 2022.

12. UK Gabapentin Study Group. Gabapentin in partial epilepsy. *Lancet* 1990;335:1114–17.

13. Electronic Medicines Compendium. *Vimpat 50mg film-coated tablets: summary of product characteristics*. Electronic Medicines Compendium, 2021. www.medicines.org.uk/emc/product/2278/smpc, last accessed 8 March 2022.

14. Electronic Medicines Compendium. *Lamotrigine 50mg tablets: summary of product characteristics*. Electronic Medicines Compendium, 2021. www.medicines.org.uk/emc/product/6092/smpc, last accessed 8 March 2022.

15. Electronic Medicines Compendium. *Levetiracetam Accord 500mg film-coated tablets: summary of product characteristics*. Electronic Medicines Compendium, 2021. www.medicines.org.uk/emc/product/7322/smpc, last accessed 8 March 2022.

16. Electronic Medicines Compendium. *Epistatus 10mg oromucosal solution: summary of product characteristics*. Electronic Medicines Compendium, 2021. www.medicines.org.uk/emc/product/2679/smpc, last accessed 8 March 2022.

17. Electronic Medicines Compendium. *Trileptal 150mg film-coated tablets: summary of product characteristics*. Electronic Medicines Compendium, 2021. www.medicines.org.uk/emc/product/3815/smpc, last accessed 8 March 2022.

18. Electronic Medicines Compendium. *Fycompa 2mg film-coated tablets: summary of product characteristics*. Electronic Medicines Compendium, 2021. www.medicines.org.uk/emc/product/4276/smpc, last accessed 8 March 2022.

19. Electronic Medicines Compendium. *Phenobarbital Accord 15mg tablets: summary of product characteristics*. Electronic Medicines Compendium, 2021. www.medicines.org.uk/emc/product/2057/smpc, last accessed 8 March 2022.

20. Electronic Medicines Compendium. *Phenytoin 100mg film-coated tablets: summary of product characteristics*. Electronic Medicines Compendium, 2022. www.medicines.org.uk/emc/medicine/26838, last accessed 8 March 2022.

21. Electronic Medicines Compendium. *Pregabalin 150mg capsules, hard: summary of product characteristics*. Electronic Medicines Compendium, 2022. www.medicines.org.uk/emc/product/7132/smpc, last accessed 8 March 2022.

22. Electronic Medicines Compendium. *Primidone SERB 50 mg tablets: summary of product characteristics*. Electronic Medicines Compendium, 2022. www.medicines.org.uk/emc/product/2941/smpc, last accessed 8 March 2022.

23. Electronic Medicines Compendium. *Inovelon 100 mg film-coated tablets: summary of product characteristics*. Electronic Medicines Compendium, 2021. www.medicines.org.uk/emc/product/410/smpc, last accessed 8 March 2022.

24. Electronic Medicines Compendium. *Sodium Valproate 200 mg gastro-resistant tablets: summary of product characteristics*. Electronic Medicines Compendium, 2020. www.medicines.org.uk/emc/product/1496/smpc, last accessed 8 March 2022.

25. Medicines and Healthcare products Regulatory Agency. *Valproate use by women and girls*. GOV.UK, 2021. www.gov.uk/guidance/valproate-use-by-women-and-girls, last accessed 4 March 2022.

26. Stephen LJ, Harden C, Tomson T, Brodie MJ. Management of epilepsy in women. *Lancet Neurol* 2019;18:481–91.

27. Electronic Medicines Compendium. *Diacomit 250 mg powder for oral suspension in sachet: summary of product characteristics*. Electronic Medicines Compendium, 2019. www.medicines.org.uk/emc/product/10304/smpc, last accessed 8 March 2022.

28. Electronic Medicines Compendium. *Gabitril 5 mg tablets: summary of product characteristics*. Electronic Medicines Compendium, 2021. www.medicines.org.uk/emc/medicine/28947, last accessed 8 March 2022.

29. Electronic Medicines Compendium. *Topiramate Accord 50 mg film-coated tablets: summary of product characteristics*. Electronic Medicines Compendium, 2021. www.medicines.org.uk/emc/product/5307/smpc, last accessed 8 March 2022.

30. Electronic Medicines Compendium. *Sabril 500 mg film-coated tablets: summary of product characteristics*. Electronic Medicines Compendium, 2021. www.medicines.org.uk/emc/product/4279/smpc, last accessed 8 March 2022.

31. Electronic Medicines Compendium. *Zonisamide Accord 100 mg hard capsules: summary of product characteristics*. Electronic Medicines Compendium, 2022. www.medicines.org.uk/emc/medicine/32938, last accessed 8 March 2022.

Further reading

National Institute for Health and Care Excellence (NICE). *Epilepsies in Children, Young People and Adults. NICE guideline [NG217]*. National Institute for Health and Care Excellence, 2022. www.nice.org.uk/guidance/ng217, last accessed 6 June 2022.

Pastalos PN. *Antiepileptic Drug Interactions: A Clinical Guide*. Clarius Press, 2005.

Shorvon S, Perucca E, Engel Jr J, eds. *The Treatment of Epilepsy*, 4th edn. Wiley Blackwell, 2015.

SIGN. *Diagnosis and Management of Epilepsy in Adults. A National Clinical Guideline*. Scottish Intercollegiate Guidelines Network, 2018. www.sign.ac.uk

6 Non-pharmacological management

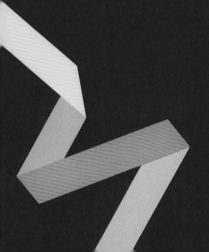

HEALTHCARE

Although pharmacological management remains the mainstay of epilepsy treatment, around 30% of people with epilepsy will continue to have seizures.[1] At a population level, this figure has remained stubbornly fixed, despite the plethora of new drugs introduced over the last 20 years or so.[2] A significant number of individuals will need an alternative, or an adjunct, to an ASM, if they are to optimize control of their seizures.

It is reasonable to consider non-ASM treatment options if good seizure control has not been achieved despite the use of two appropriate drugs given at optimal doses. Surgery should be the first consideration in these circumstances because it offers the best chance of complete, or substantially improved, long-term seizure control.[3] This is particularly true if local investigations have identified a seizure focus, but even in the absence of imaging abnormalities, referral to a tertiary center offering epilepsy surgery should be considered for adults with focal-onset seizures.

Epilepsy surgery

Surgery for seizures falls into three distinct subsets:
- resective procedures (potentially curative)
- disconnective procedures (usually palliative)
- implantable stimulators (usually palliative).

Surgical resection involves identifying the epileptogenic focus and removing it. Disconnective approaches interfere with epileptogenic circuitry to limit the spread of neuronal discharges across the cortex, while implantable stimulators work by modulating epileptogenic circuitry, for example the limbic system. Surgical outcomes are generally recorded using the ILAE outcome classification scale (Table 6.1),[4] while the choice of surgical procedure will depend on the indication (Table 6.2).

Presurgical evaluation. Standards have been published governing the operation of an epilepsy surgery center.[5] However, there is no universally agreed protocol to identify potential surgical candidates.[6] Presurgical evaluation aims to establish the presence of drug resistance, delineate the epileptogenic zone to be resected and demonstrate that its removal will not cause additional unacceptable neurological or

TABLE 6.1

ILAE surgical outcome classification scales[4]

Classification	Outcome
Class I	Seizure free; no auras
Class II	Auras only
Class III	1–3 seizure days per year ± auras
Class IV	4 seizure days per year to 50% reduction in baseline seizure days ± auras
Class V	<50% reduction in baseline number of seizure days to 100% increase in baseline number of seizure days ± auras
Class VI	>100% increase in baseline number of seizure days ± auras

TABLE 6.2

Types of epilepsy surgery and their indications

Procedure	Indication
Anterior temporal lobectomy	Mesial temporal sclerosis
Focal resection	Focal-onset seizures arising from resectable cortex
Corpus callosotomy	Tonic, atonic or tonic–clonic seizures, with falling and injury; large non-resectable lesions; secondary bilateral synchrony
Hemispherectomy	Rasmussen's syndrome or other unilateral hemisphere pathology in association with functionally impaired contralateral hand
Subpial transections	Partial-onset seizures arising from unresectable cortex

cognitive deficits. In practice, the evaluation involves the following processes.

- A thorough review of the patient's seizure history and ASM trials.
- Sophisticated video-EEG monitoring, which localizes the onset of several seizures that are typical for the patient.
- High-quality MRI with a dedicated 'epilepsy surgery protocol' to increase diagnostic accuracy.
- Functional imaging such as SPECT or PET, when necessary, to delineate a potential epileptogenic zone.
- Neuropsychological testing, including intracarotid injection of amobarbital or functional MRI, to define the laterality of language and memory functions.

Lobar excision may be carried out with a high probability of improvement when all the following are satisfied.

- EEG monitoring shows that seizure onset is consistently and repeatedly from the same portion of one frontal or temporal lobe.
- Other investigations are consistent with this localization.
- The identified area can be removed safely without permanent cognitive, sensory or motor deficit.

If scalp EEG data do not clearly identify the seizure focus, or if the neuroimaging and/or neuropsychological testing results are inconsistent with the ictal findings, 'invasive' electrodes may be inserted into the brain for further seizure recording, often guided by the results of functional neuroimaging (Figures 6.1–6.3). When monitoring shows that seizures arise from different sides of the brain on separate occasions, or are consistent with generalized seizures, lobectomy is unlikely to be of benefit. Intracranial electrodes also facilitate 'mapping' of eloquent cortex (areas with important functions such as motor and speech) so that it may be avoided during subsequent resection. Advances in neuroimaging techniques are reducing the need for invasive intracranial EEG recording.

Resective surgery. The most common resective procedure is anterior temporal lobectomy for hippocampal or mesial temporal sclerosis. In well-selected cases, 70–80% of patients can become seizure free, with a surgical mortality close to 0% and less than 5% significant morbidity (for example, hemiparesis, hemianopia). Some patients may be suitable candidates for a more limited resection known as

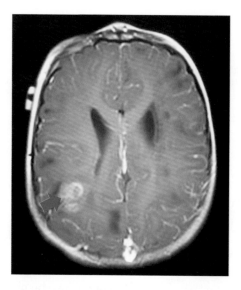

Figure 6.1 MRI scan of a patient with refractory epilepsy showing a heterogeneous lesion in the right parietal lobe (arrow).

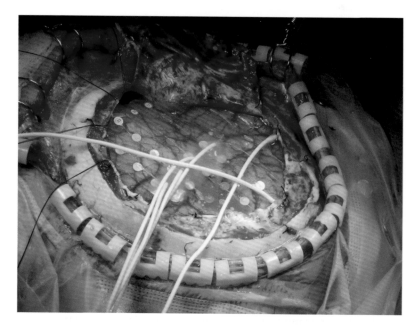

Figure 6.2 EEG electrodes applied to the cortical surface over the lesion intraoperatively to map out the area to be resected.

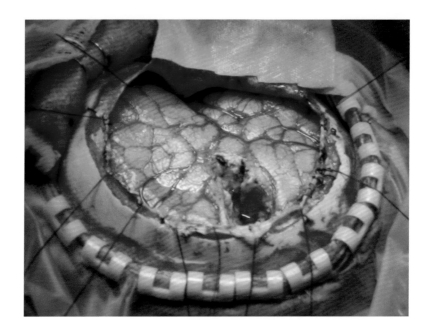

Figure 6.3 Patient in Figure 6.2 immediately after focal resection of the cortical lesion.

amygdalohippocampectomy in which the epileptogenic hippocampus and amygdala are removed, while sparing the temporal neocortex. Other potentially curative procedures include lesionectomy to resect discrete structural lesions such as glial tumors and vascular malformations.

Disconnective surgery. These procedures include hemispherectomy/ functional hemispherectomy, corpus callosotomy and multiple subpial transection. The focus of the seizure is not resected. Instead, the aim is to disrupt the pathways that are important for the spread of epileptiform discharges to reduce the frequency and severity of seizures. Corpus callosotomy is an option for patients with severe generalized epilepsy, particularly atonic seizures, with frequent falls and subsequent injuries. Multiple subpial transection is performed when the epileptogenic lesion cannot be removed because of its proximity to eloquent cortex, although it has more recently fallen out of favor as it offers limited benefit. Hemispherectomy is a more drastic procedure in which an extensively diseased and epileptogenic cerebral hemisphere is removed or left in place but functionally disconnected from other brain structures.

Vagus nerve stimulation (VNS), since its introduction in 1994, has arguably become the first-choice treatment for patients with drug-resistant epilepsy who are not suitable for other types of surgery, or for whom other surgical procedures have failed to produce adequate benefits.

The VNS system consists of a programmable signal generator implanted in the patient's left upper chest. Bipolar leads connect the generator to the left vagus nerve in the neck (Figure 6.4). Stimulation is configured using a programming wand, which non-invasively communicates with the signal generator. A handheld magnet can be used by the patient or carer to provide additional stimulation in the presence of seizure triggers or at the onset of a seizure, to limit its severity. Newer devices incorporate autostimulation based on changes

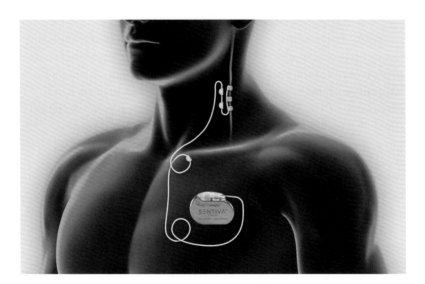

Figure 6.4 VNS system in which the VNS pulse generator is linked by electrodes to the left vagus nerve in the neck. The ends of the flexible silicone leads are wrapped around the nerve. Reproduced courtesy of LivaNova, Texas, USA.

in heart rate that occur at the onset of a seizure, with the aim of aborting it.

The VNS device is generally turned on a couple of weeks after implantation. Stimulation is then titrated, in terms of signal frequency and 'on time' versus 'off time', according to clinical effect and tolerability. Optimal effects are usually only seen after many months, or even a couple of years, following implantation.

Mechanism of action. The mechanism by which VNS exerts its antiseizure properties is multifactorial.[7] Action potentials generated at the cathode (negative electrode) travel afferently along the vagus nerve to the brainstem. Efferent action potentials are mainly blocked by the positive electrode, thereby reducing potential side effects. Most vagal afferent synapses end in the nucleus tractus solitarius (NTS) of the brainstem. Stimulation of the NTS has been shown to increase GABA signaling or decrease glutamate signaling. The NTS has major projections to the locus coeruleus (LC), the dorsal raphe nuclei (DRN) and the parabrachial nucleus (PBN). VNS increases resting-state autonomous firing of the LC and DRN. Stimulation of the LC suppresses epileptic activity within the amygdala.

The LC and the DRN are, respectively, the main noradrenaline and serotonin production sites in the brain, and stimulation of these areas may account for the antidepressant effects of VNS (and the higher serotonin metabolites found in the cerebrospinal fluid of patients who receive VNS). The NTS also has direct connections to the limbic system via the amygdala and thalamus. VNS has been shown to prevent the lowering of seizure thresholds of neurons in the amygdala as well as potentially decreasing excitability and thereby seizure generation in the hippocampus. There are reciprocal connections between the prefrontal cortex and the brainstem, thalamus, basal ganglia and limbic system.

Therapeutic responses to VNS are associated with increased $GABA_A$ receptor density in cortical regions. VNS has an acute antiseizure effect: responsive VNS uses cardiac cues to deliver a train of stimulations close to seizure onset, which may shorten or stop the seizure by containing its propagation. After responsive VNS treatment, seizures are more localized or lateralized to a smaller portion of the brain. However, chronic stimulation also seems to have an antiepileptogenic effect, as seizures are less frequent and, indeed, have a less severe clinical semiology.

Tolerability. Serious adverse events are rare and are mainly surgery related. These can include infection, nerve paralysis, facial paresis and left vocal cord paralysis. Voice alteration (hoarseness) and coughing are the most common non-serious adverse events, affecting approximately half of patients in clinical trials, with a wide range of severity.[8] In practice, the device is generally very well tolerated, and patients become accustomed to the stimulation. The handheld magnet can be strapped across the device to temporarily turn off stimulation, for example, if the patient has a sore throat or needs to make a public speech.

Combined data from clinical trials suggest that around one-third of patients can expect a 50% reduction in seizure frequency by using the device.[8] However, these trials were conducted over 12 weeks. In clinical practice, results are much more encouraging. A recent case series reported 59% of patients with a greater than 50% reduction in seizure frequency. Additionally, a further cohort of patients were switched to the new Aspire SR model from their existing device. The first device produced a 50% or greater seizure reduction for 53% of patients. When they were switched to the Aspire SR, 71% of those patients reported a further 50% or greater reduction in their seizure burden.[9] A small number of patients may become completely seizure free.

Direct electrical brain stimulation. There are currently two direct brain stimulation systems available for the treatment of epilepsy, deep-brain stimulation (DBS) and responsive neural stimulation (RNS). DBS is an open-loop neurostimulator that provides continuous, periodic electrical stimulation to suppress seizures. RNS is a closed-loop neurostimulator that automatically analyzes electrocortical activity to detect the onset of epileptiform activity and rapidly deliver electrical stimulation to terminate the seizure.[10] In common with VNS, both systems require a prolonged programming period to achieve optimal effects.

As the name suggests, DBS involves the implantation of electrodes directly into cortical tissue. The stimulation will only have a local effect, so placement of the electrodes is very important. RNS electrodes tend to be implanted within or close to the epileptogenic focus, typically the hippocampus. DBS electrodes are usually implanted into the anterior nucleus of the thalamus. Although other locations have been used, there is currently insufficient evidence to support their general clinical use.[10]

All forms of electrical brain stimulation show improved efficacy over time. This has led to suggestions that the stimulation may provide disease modification benefits as well as seizure suppression, and possibly seizure termination (Figure 6.5). However, there

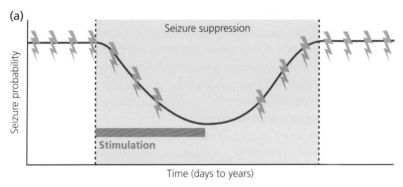

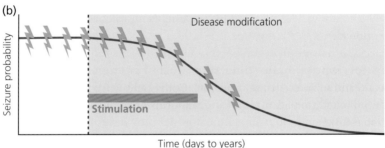

Figure 6.5 Representation of chronic effects of neurostimulation. (a) In established epilepsy, seizure suppression (shaded region) temporarily reduces the probability of seizures, with no permanent effect on disease state of epilepsy. (b) In established epilepsy, disease modification (shaded region) results in permanent reduction in seizure frequency, ideally resulting in seizure freedom or 'cure', even after stimulation is stopped. The solid bar in each graph represents the duration of stimulation. Adapted from Foutz and Wong 2021.[10]

are several confounding factors. As discussed above, technology continues to improve, as do programming techniques, which could account for additional benefits. For RNS it is unclear whether improvements in seizure control are due to seizure suppression or to termination of seizures immediately after onset and before they clinically manifest. Nevertheless, all forms of stimulation seem to offer benefit, with progressive and sustained seizure reduction over several years.

Dietary approaches

Ketogenic diet. Fasting has long been recognized as a way to control seizures. In the early 1900s, several studies demonstrated the short-term benefits of fasting, which led to the discovery that ketones were produced by the liver in otherwise healthy people when they were starved or if they consumed a very-low-carbohydrate, high-fat diet.[11] The original ketogenic diet used 1 g of protein per kilogram of bodyweight in children, 10–15 g of carbohydrates per day with the remainder of calories made up from fat. Though relatively successful, particularly in children, the diet fell out of favor, partly because of the introduction of new ASM and partly because it was extremely unpalatable. Dieticians have since been creative with menus to make the modern ketogenic diet more palatable.

Although still largely used in children, there are some centers worldwide that offer treatment to adults. All individuals will require specialist monitoring from clinicians familiar with the diet. Some epilepsy syndromes are particularly suited to a ketogenic diet, such as DS and seizures arising from TSC. Conversely, the presence of certain conditions contraindicates all forms of ketogenic diet therapy (Table 6.3).[12]

The original ketogenic diet used a ratio of four portions of fat to one portion of protein plus carbohydrates, known as the 4:1. The modified Atkins diet utilizes a 1:1 ratio of fat to carbohydrates and protein. It does not entail weighing food, or restriction of calories, protein or liquids. This makes it more flexible and suitable for adolescents and adults. Nevertheless, carbohydrates are still severely restricted, generally to 15–20 g per day.

Seizure reduction and adherence to the diet is lower in adults and adolescents than children. A recent meta-analysis examined patients

TABLE 6.3

Absolute contraindications to the use of ketogenic diet therapies

- Carnitine deficiency (primary)
- Carnitine palmitoyltransferase I or II deficiency
- Carnitine translocase deficiency
- β-oxidation defects
- Medium-chain acyl dehydrogenase deficiency
- Long-chain acyl dehydrogenase deficiency
- Short-chain acyl dehydrogenase deficiency
- Long-chain 3-hydroxyacyl-CoA deficiency
- Medium-chain 3-hydroxyacyl-CoA deficiency
- Pyruvate carboxylase deficiency
- Porphyria

Reproduced from Kossoff et al.[12] Optimal clinical management of children receiving dietary therapies for epilepsy: Updated recommendations of the International Ketogenic Diet Study Group

aged 15–86 years with treatment times ranging from 3–36 months: 20–70% of patients had a greater than 50% seizure reduction, with seizure freedom ranges of 7–30%. Discontinuation rates varied from 12.5–82%.[13]

Low glycemic index diet. This diet uses a ratio of 0.6:1 fat to carbohydrates and protein. Efficacy seems very good, but most reports are of small case series with poor methodology. Most studies have concerned children, although some adults have reported benefits. Interestingly, there have been reports of ongoing improvements in seizure control after discontinuation of the diet, perhaps suggesting an element of disease modification.[14]

Complementary (not alternative) treatments

A wide variety of non-pharmacological non-surgical approaches have been suggested for people with epilepsy. These complementary treatments will almost universally be used alongside other forms of treatment, mainly ASM. Therefore, 'complementary treatment' is a much better term than 'alternative therapy', as it is unlikely that the patient will be able to substitute these therapies for medication (though a reduction in drug burden may be possible), and to do so, in most cases, would be deleterious to their care.

A large body of evidence has been produced to show that complementary treatments can be beneficial for some people with epilepsy. However, there are methodological limitations to most of the published studies. It is often difficult to be certain whether participants have epilepsy, PNES, or a combination of the two, and many complementary techniques will be helpful to patients with both conditions. The relationship between the patient and therapist is also important, making it difficult to generalize some of the study outcomes.

Most complementary treatments are reported as case studies or have involved trials with very limited numbers of participants. Most authors report the outcome of a single intervention, rather than an attempt to use multiple techniques to help individuals take control of their seizures. An exception is the Andrews/Reiter Epilepsy Research Program. This clinic uses stepwise methods, set out in a workbook format, utilizing trained epilepsy counsellors to guide individuals toward self-control of their epilepsy. A small sample of the several thousand people treated using the program suggested that half had a greater than 50% reduction in seizures, with 37% becoming seizure free at the end of the program.[15] However, the resources of most health economies are such that a comprehensive program will not readily be available. An algorithm for the complementary treatment of epilepsy was proposed some years ago, and it remains helpful to consider this stepwise approach.[16]

Different approaches will resonate with different patients, making a 'one-size-fits-all' approach problematic at best and potentially counterproductive. What is offered to patients will be heavily dependent upon local resources and the interests of individual clinicians.

Basic approaches include seizure triggers, lifestyle choices, adherence to medication and patient education (Table 6.4). Wolf and Okujava coined the term 'life hygiene' to describe the process.[17] Careful

TABLE 6.4.

Basic approaches to cover with all patients at, or soon after, diagnosis

- Discussion of general triggers
  - Alcohol/illicit drugs
  - Prescribed medication that can alter the seizure threshold
  - Stress/anxiety
  - Diet (regular meals and avoidance of excitotoxins)
  - Sleep deprivation
- Discussion of specific triggers individual to the patient
- Medically based 'what is epilepsy' session
- Adherence to ASM

evaluation of individual factors precipitating the first seizure(s), and subsequent avoidance of these factors, can be highly effective. Any member of the healthcare team can address these issues and this simple intervention can often be successful in reducing the frequency of seizures.

Unfortunately, many patients leave their consultations believing that ASM will stop their seizures without the need to modify their lifestyle. They are then surprised if this proves not to be the case. Moreover, patients may not be concordant with their medication. Deliberate avoidance, for reasons ranging from unwanted side effects to material gain from ongoing seizures, or genuine forgetfulness, remembering that epilepsy can have a detrimental effect on short-term memory, are the most common reasons. Seizure reductions of up to 50% have been reported following educational programs addressing the importance of following prescribed ASM regimens.

Intermediate approaches. Neurobehavioral therapy is an attempt to prevent seizures by interrupting the sequence of events leading up to them. It highlights the importance of exploring the emotional life of the patient at seizure onset. This information is often overlooked by treating physicians. Behaviors and psychological variables can have a huge impact on clinical conditions, pathophysiology and even the effectiveness of pharmacological agents. Growing evidence suggests a bidirectional interaction between the presence of seizures and psychological states.

There is considerable overlap in the possible psychological approaches for the treatment of seizures due to epilepsy and those caused by PNES (see Chapter 10). High levels of emotion are the most common psychological seizure triggers. Negative emotions such as conflict, fear, pressure to perform and rage are commonly described, but any heightened emotion, for example, excitement (often seen in patients who have ID), can be a trigger. Another feature is the unfavorable response to an aura, making a full-blown seizure more likely.

Physiological reactions may involve over-breathing and exhibited fear, not only of the seizure itself, but also of the embarrassment that accompanies it. This seizure phobia is a recently documented phenomenon that affects people with epilepsy and PNES, has a female predominance and is associated with anxiety disorder and past major depression.[18] Adequately treating depression may improve seizure control. Antidepressants can sometimes trigger seizures (though they are not contraindicated), but psychological therapies have been shown to be effective, particularly those with a mindfulness-based approach.[19,20]

Sometimes patients develop countermeasures to abort or postpone seizures. For example, someone with seizures incorporating a Jacksonian march may be able to prevent seizure spread by holding the affected arm above the point that it is jerking and concentrating hard on stopping the seizure. There are also documented cases of women managing to postpone a seizure until they got their children to a place of safety.

Advanced approaches. There is some fluidity between intermediate and advanced approaches. For example, utilizing some forms of mindfulness could be considered intermediate, whereas a full program based on acceptance commitment therapy (ACT) or mindfulness-based cognitive therapy[20] would require advanced skills. These behavioral techniques aim to internalize the patient's locus of control to empower them to establish subjective management of their seizures. Cognitive behavioral therapy (CBT), whereby patients learn to identify unhelpful thought traits and establish alternative cognitive and behavioral responses to enhance emotional well-being, is undoubtedly the most widely used technique, but intuitively, ACT, with its emphasis on accepting difficult memories and situations, while focusing on what is important and life enhancing, may resonate better with many patients.

Generic stress reduction techniques, such as relaxation and breathing exercises, are widely used alongside other psychobehavioral approaches. Other intensive programs, based on relaxation, have been tried with some reported successes. A trial in the UK showed benefits of aromatherapy, particularly in combination with hypnotherapy, in the treatment of seizures.[21] Several studies from India demonstrated significant seizure improvements in patients practicing Sahaj yoga compared with a control group using a sham technique.[22]

Diet-based therapies also constitute advanced approaches (see above).

Specialized approaches. The concept of interrupting seizure progression has been taken one stage further by the advocates of biofeedback. Seizure thresholds change in relation to certain EEG rhythms. The most important factor in the successful use of EEG biofeedback is the ability of participants to achieve awareness and control of different brainwave patterns. Seminal work by Sterman[23] using operant conditioning concludes that 'this must be a simple skill, as cats seem quite competent in this regard...!' EEG biofeedback uses relaxation techniques to teach people to achieve 8–14 Hz alpha rhythm, an EEG pattern that is incompatible with seizures. This approach is expensive in terms of the equipment needed and the expertise required. However, it may be the most promising of the behavioral approaches, with up to 74% of patients reporting fewer seizures following training.[20]

Herbal remedies: a warning

In the authors' experience, there is no role for herbal remedies in the treatment of epilepsy. Indeed, they can be detrimental as some patients may stop taking ASM in favor of these remedies. Nevertheless, many people with epilepsy do take herbal and/or dietary supplements (for example, St John's wort for depression or valerian for difficulty sleeping), so it is important to initiate discussion about their current and/or intended use of these products. Sometimes, this can provide helpful clues to the side effects and comorbidities the patient is experiencing, but also ensures appropriate advice is given about possible herb–ASM interactions, including effects on seizure frequency and serum ASM concentrations. For example, St John's wort can affect hepatic metabolism and therefore alter the serum concentrations of hepatically metabolized ASM. In addition, there are anecdotal reports to suggest that some essential oils, evening primrose and borage, and stimulants such as ephdra (ma huang) and guarana may exacerbate seizures.[24]

 Key points – non-pharmacological management

- Non-ASM approaches can be considered if good seizure control has not been achieved despite the use of two drugs at optimal doses.
- Surgery offers the best chance of complete, or substantially improved, long-term seizure control.
- VNS has become the first-choice approach in individuals with drug-resistant epilepsy who are not suitable for other surgical options.
- Progressive and sustained reductions in seizure burden can be achieved with electrical brain stimulation.
- Individuals following a ketogenic diet to help control their seizures require specialist monitoring.
- Complementary treatments may be beneficial in some people with epilepsy but are unlikely to replace the need for ASM.
- EEG biofeedback, while a specialized non-pharmaceutical strategy for seizure management, appears to be a promising behavioral approach.
- People with epilepsy may be interested in using herbal supplements to alleviate side effects from ASM but such use should be carefully discussed with their physician as certain ASM have significant interactions with many supplements.

References

1. Kwan P, Brodie MJ. Early identification of refractory epilepsy. *N Engl J Med* 2000;342:314–19.

2. Blond BN, Hirsch LJ, Mattson RH. Misperceptions on the chance of seizure freedom with antiseizure medications after two failed trials. *Epilepsia* 2020;61:1789–90.

3. Mohan M, Keller S, Nicolson A et al. *The long-term outcomes of epilepsy surgery. PLoS One* 2018;13:e0196274.

4. Weiser HG, Blume WT, Fish D et al. ILAE commission report. Proposal for a new classification of outcome with respect to epileptic seizures following epilepsy surgery. *Epilepsia* 2001;42:282–6.

5. Rosenow F, Bast T, Czech T et al. Revised version of quality guidelines for presurgical epilepsy evaluation and surgical epilepsy therapy issued by the Austrian, German, and Swiss working group on presurgical epilepsy diagnosis and operative epilepsy treatment. *Epilepsia* 2016;57:1215–20.

6. Ghaffari-Rafi A, Leon-Rojas J. Investigatory pathway and principles of patient selection for epilepsy surgery candidates: a systematic review. *BMC Neurol* 2020;20:100.

7. Schachter SC, Garcia P, Dashe JF. Vagus nerve stimulation therapy for the treatment of epilepsy. UpToDate, 2022. www.uptodate.com/contents/vagus-nerve-stimulation-therapy-for-the-treatment-of-epilepsy/print, last accessed 11 April 2022.

8. LivaNova. *VNS Therapy® System Epilepsy Physician's Manual.* LivaNova, 2021. https://dynamic.cyberonics.com/manuals/emanual_download.asp?lang=English-US&docid={BAA7EE19-92D5-4E78-8480-5BB49CD87744}, last accessed 4 March 2022.

9. Hamilton P, Soryal I, Dhahri P et al. Clinical outcomes of VNS therapy with AspireSR® (including cardiac-based seizure detection) at a large complex epilepsy and surgery centre. *Seizure* 2018;58:120–6.

10. Foutz T, Wong M. Brain stimulation treatments and epilepsy: basic mechanisms and clinical advances. *Biomed J* 2021;S2319-4170(21)00110-4.

11. Wheless JW. History and origin of the ketogenic diet. In: Stafstrom CE, Rho JM, eds. *Epilepsy and the Ketogenic Diet.* Springer, 2004:31–50.

12. Kossoff EH, Zupec-Kania BA, Auvin S et al. Optimal clinical management of children receiving dietary therapies for epilepsy: updated recommendations of the International Ketogenic Diet Study Group. *Epilepsia Open* 2018;3:175–92.

13. Liu H, Yang Y, Wang Y et al. Ketogenic diet for treatment of intractable epilepsy in adults: a meta-analysis of observational studies. *Epilepsia Open* 2018;3:9–17.

14. D'Andrea Meira I, Romão TT, Pires do Prado HJ et al. Ketogenic diet and epilepsy: what we know so far. *Front Neurosci* 2019;13:5.

15. Michaelis R, Schonfeld W, Elas SM. Trigger self-control and seizure arrest in the Andrews/Reiter behavioural approach to epilepsy: a retrospective analysis of seizure frequency. *Epilepsy Behav* 2012;23:266–71.

16. Tittensor PA. To treat and how to treat: an algorithm of alternative methods of seizure control. *Epilepsy Care* 2005;1:6–9.

17. Wolf P, Okujava N. Possibilities of non-pharmacological conservative treatment of epilepsy. *Seizure* 1999;8:45–52.

18. Weiss A, Canetti L, David SB et al. Seizure phobia: a distinct psychiatric disorder among people with epilepsy. *Seizure* 2022;95:26–32.

19. Thompson NJ, McGee RE, Garcia-Williams A et al. The impact of a depression self-management intervention on seizure activity. *Epilepsy Behav* 2020;103:106504.

20. Tang V, Michaelis R, Kwan P. Psychobehavioural therapy for epilepsy. *Epilepsy Behav* 2014;32:147–55.

21. Betts T. Use of aromatherapy (with or without hypnosis) in the treatment of intractable epilepsy – a two-year follow-up study. *Seizure* 2003;12:534–8.

22. Yardi N. Yoga for control of epilepsy. *Seizure* 2001;10:7–12.

23. Sterman MB. Sensorimotor EEG feedback training in the study and treatment of epilepsy. In: Mostofsky DI, Loyning Y, eds. *The Neurobehavioural Treatment of Epilepsy.* Psychology Press, 1993.

24. Samuels N, Finkelstein Y, Singer SR, Oberbaum M. Herbal medicine and epilepsy: proconvulsive effects and interactions with antiepileptic drugs. *Epilepsia* 2008;49:373–80.

7 Status epilepticus and seizure clusters

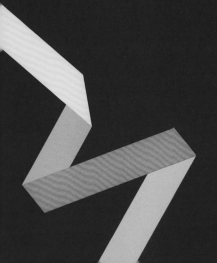

HEALTHCARE

Status epilepticus

SE is a life-threatening medical emergency that results from either of the following.

- Failure of the mechanisms required for a seizure to stop.
- The initiation of mechanisms that lead to seizures being abnormally prolonged.[1]

Initiating emergency treatment in a timely manner improves the chances of terminating a seizure early and minimizing adverse events and long-term consequences, including neuronal death, neuronal injury and change to neuronal networks.

The time point at which a seizure is unlikely to self-terminate is defined as T_1. T_1 varies according to seizure type:

- 5 minutes for tonic–clonic SE
- 10 minutes for focal impaired-awareness SE
- 10–15 minutes for absence SE.[1]

Time point T_2 is when neuronal injury can occur. This is 30 minutes from seizure onset for tonic–clonic SE and beyond 60 minutes for focal impaired-awareness SE.[1] There are insufficient data to establish T_1 or T_2 for other seizure types.

Focal-onset and GTCS that spontaneously self-terminate within 3 minutes do not need emergency treatment (see Chapter 9 for first aid management).

Types of status epilepticus. The most readily recognized type of SE is convulsive. This presents as focal-onset and/or GTCS and is associated with the highest morbidity and mortality risk. Non-convulsive SE (NCSE) accounts for 20–30% of SE[2] and diagnosis can only be established by concurrent EEG recording. NCSE includes focal aware motor SE with motor seizures localized to one side of the body, known as epilepsia partiallis continua. NCSE without prominent motor phenomena include focal impaired-awareness SE, focal impaired-cognitive SE and absence SE.

Causes. Acute symptomatic causes account for up to 60% of SE in adults without a previous diagnosis of epilepsy. SE can occur within 7 days of an acute event (for example, stroke, intoxication, infection), after 7 days for other remote symptomatic causes (for example, brain injury, encephalitis) and in association with symptomatic progressive causes (brain neoplasm, dementia, etc.). Triggers include sleep deprivation, lack of adherence to ASM, low ASM plasma concentrations, alcohol withdrawal and underlying brain pathology.[3] Other possible acute or chronic processes that risk causing SE are outlined in Table 7.1, as well as differential diagnoses, most notably PNES.[4]

TABLE 7.1

Causes of status epilepticus

Acute processes
- CNS infections (meningitis, encephalitis, intracranial abscess)
- Metabolic abnormalities (hypoglycemia, hyponatremia, hypocalcemia, hepatic encephalopathy)
- Cerebrovascular accidents
- Head trauma (with or without intracranial bleed)
- Drug toxicity
- Drug withdrawal syndromes (e.g. alcohol, benzodiazepines, barbiturates)
- Hypoxia
- Hypertensive emergency
- Autoimmune disorders

Chronic processes
- Pre-existing epilepsy with breakthrough seizures
- Non-adherence to ASM
- Alcohol withdrawal
- CNS tumors
- Remote CNS pathology (e.g. traumatic brain injury, stroke)

Differential diagnosis
- Acute intoxication
- Early catastrophic brain hypoxia
- Encephalopathy of toxic and metabolic origin
- Ischemic stroke
- PNES
- Trauma

Adapted from Wylie et al. 2021.[4]

Mortality/morbidity. The incidence of SE varies worldwide, ranging from 10–40 per 100000 people per year, with a mortality rate in adults of approximately 30% and up to 40% in those with drug-resistant SE.[3] Other studies of long-term outcomes by age have reported mortality rates of 22% in children with SE and 57% in adults.[5] Mortality and morbidity reflect the underlying cause and the physiological effects of SE, including hypertension, tachycardia, cardiac arrhythmias and hyperthermia. Mortality is higher when SE is secondary to an acute insult (such as acute stroke, anoxia, trauma, infections and metabolic disturbance). Conversely, SE resulting from a previous stroke, excessive alcohol or alcohol withdrawal or ASM withdrawal has a more favorable prognosis.

Management. A long duration of SE is associated with poor outcome. An effective management protocol should therefore be initiated immediately. Any delay in treatment worsens the prognosis and reduces the likelihood of stopping seizures without having to resort to general anesthesia.[6]

0–5 minutes: initial management in the community setting. When a person with or without epilepsy experiences their first prolonged tonic–clonic seizure and/or repeated tonic–clonic seizures in the community, the emergency services should be called immediately for early intervention. Some people with epilepsy who have experienced SE previously will already have an emergency ASM, such as oromucosal midazolam (or rectal diazepam if oromucosal midazolam is contraindicated or unavailable), and an agreed treatment plan for family, friends and/or caregivers to follow. Having received approved basic epilepsy and safe-rescue medication administration training,[7] family, friends and/or caregivers will know how to administer rescue medication up to 5 minutes from the onset of the seizure and to call the emergency services if the seizure does not terminate within 10 minutes. They will also have learnt how to protect the person from injury and prevent aspiration until help arrives.

0–5 minutes: initial management in the hospital setting. A clinical guideline and treatment algorithm for the management of adults with prolonged seizures and/or tonic–clonic SE in a hospital setting is shown in Appendix 1 (page 197).[8]

Emergency management should be initiated as soon as a tonic–clonic seizure begins and SE is confirmed (T_1). The patient should be placed in a semiprone position with their head down to prevent aspiration. Oxygen should be administered with continuous monitoring of respiration, pulse, blood pressure and temperature. A 12-lead ECG should be obtained. Gaining intravenous access will allow blood sampling for metabolic studies, a toxin screen and assessment of ASM levels (for people being treated for epilepsy), blood gases and blood glucose. Hypoglycemia, suspicions of excess alcohol, infections or electrolyte imbalances should be treated accordingly.

Potential acute and chronic causes of SE should be investigated and neuroimaging and EEG considered if appropriate. Gathering the epilepsy and ASM history for individuals with diagnosed epilepsy can help determine whether SE has resulted from a recent change to their ASM, poor adherence or alterations in ASM plasma concentration. It is also important to consider differential diagnosis and the possibility of PNES.

T_1 *5–15 minutes (early status): first-line treatment.* The patient should be treated with a first dose of intravenous lorazepam, oromucosal midazolam or rectal diazepam if oromucosal midazolam is unavailable, with a second dose administered after 5 minutes if the seizure has not stopped (see Appendix 1 for dose information). Intramuscular midazolam is an option if oral/and or rectal administration is contraindicated or unavailable.

15 minutes onwards (established status): second-line treatment. Patients who do not respond to first-line treatment must be elevated to critical care level and an anesthetist contacted. A third dose of ASM (LEV, fosphenytoin or PHT, or VPA [see Appendix 1 for dose information]) should be administered. As no difference in efficacy or adverse events has been established for these drugs, choice of ASM should be guided by type of epilepsy, sex, ASM history, comorbidities and other drug interactions.[8] However, if SE has been caused by non-adherence, the patient's usual ASM (if available as an intravenous formulation) may be the best choice. Cardiac and blood pressure monitoring should be maintained during infusion because of the risk of extravasation and phlebitis.

Loading doses of each ASM vary according to bodyweight: for example, in a 70kg patient, PHT loading would take 28 minutes, LEV 10 minutes and VPA 5 minutes at the recommended rates. If the seizure has not stopped after the infusion, the process should be repeated using another of the above drugs. PB can also be considered (see Appendix 1).

T_2 *30 minutes onwards: third-line (drug-resistant status) and fourth-line (super-resistant status) treatment.* Seizures lasting more than 30 minutes from onset are defined as drug resistant; those lasting more than 24 hours are defined as super-resistant. Patients should be transferred to an intensive care unit 60–90 minutes after seizure onset, and supervised by an anesthetist and healthcare professionals qualified to induce and maintain general anesthesia and airway and cardiac support (see Appendix 1).

Seizure clusters

Some people with severe and poorly controlled epilepsy experience clusters of seizures lasting from minutes to hours. Seizure clusters have also been variably defined as at least three seizures in 24 hours, at least two seizures in 24 hours and at least two seizures in 6 hours.[9] Patients with frontal lobe epilepsy are particularly prone to clustering of seizures at night. Seizure clustering may occur around menstruation in women, or when a person does not take their usual ASM. In most cases, however, precipitating factors cannot be readily identified. These seizure clusters may not be defined as SE but nonetheless require therapeutic intervention to prevent SE and admission to the emergency department. Acute treatment with a benzodiazepine such as CLB after the first seizure can be given to try to prevent further attacks. If the seizure cluster is a result of ASM omission or dose reduction, reintroduction of the drug may be sufficient to abort it.

Key points – status epilepticus and seizure clusters

- SE is a life-threatening medical emergency.
- SE can be convulsive or non-convulsive.
- Emergency treatment should be given when a focal-onset or GTCS has lasted up to 5 minutes.
- Poor prognostic factors for SE include older age, an acute symptomatic cause and long duration.
- Benzodiazepine administration can be useful in patients experiencing clusters of seizures.
- CAUTION: not all seizures are epileptic and accurate diagnosis of SE is vital! In PNES, treatment with sedation or ASM is detrimental.

Key references

1. Trinka E, Cock H, Hesdorffer D et al. A definition and classification of status epilepticus – report of the ILAE Task Force on classification of status epilepticus. *Epilepsia* 2015;56:1515–23.

2. García-Villafranca A, Barrera-López L, Pose-Bar M et al. De-novo non-convulsive status epilepticus in adult medical inpatients without known epilepsy: analysis of mortality related factors and literature review. *PLoS One* 2021;16:e0258602.

3. Ascoli M, Ferlazzo E, Gasparini S et al. Epidemiology and outcomes of status epilepticus. *Int J Gen Med* 2021;14:2965–73.

4. Wylie T, Sandhu DS, Murr N. *Status Epilepticus*. In: StatPearls [Internet], 2021. www.ncbi.nlm. nih.gov/books/NBK430686, last accessed 4 March 2022.

5. Sculier C, Gaínza-Lein M, Sánchez Fernández I, Loddenkemper T. Long-term outcomes of status epilepticus: a critical assessment. *Epilepsia* 2018;59:155–69.

6. Glauser T, Shinnar S, Gloss D et al. Evidence-based guideline: treatment of convulsive status epilepticus in children and adults: report of the guideline committee of the American Epilepsy Society. *Epilepsy Curr* 2016;16:48–61.

7. Tittensor P, Tittensor S, Chisanga E et al. UK framework for basic epilepsy training and oromucosal midazolam administration. *Epilepsy Behav* 2021;122:108180.

8. Mitchell J, Adan G, Whitehead C et al. *Status Epilepticus Guideline.* The Walton Centre NHS Foundation Trust, 2020. www.thewaltoncentre.nhs.uk/ Downloads/Information%20 for%20healthcare%20 professionals/Status%20 Epilepticus%20Guidelines%20 July%202020.pdf, last accessed 4 March 2022.

9. Jafarpour S, Hirsch LJ, Gaínza-Lein M et al. Seizure cluster: definition, prevalence, consequences, and management. *Seizure* 2019;68:9–15.

8 Specific populations

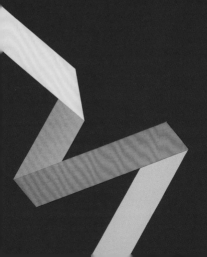

HEALTHCARE

Girls and women of childbearing age

All girls and women with epilepsy should receive individualized accurate advice and information about contraception, menstruation, pregnancy, breastfeeding and caring for infants. This needs to be given at regular intervals by nurses, pharmacists and other allied healthcare professionals so teenage girls and women with epilepsy can make informed decisions about their epilepsy management and reproductive health.

Contraception. Hepatic enzyme-inducing ASM can cause some contraceptives to fail (Table 8.1). The metabolism of ASM can alter the menstrual cycle and increase turnover of the components of OCPs and depot formulations of steroid hormones.

To be effective, the combined OCP must provide at least 50 µg of estrogen/day. Medroxyprogesterone depot injections appear to be effective, and a levonorgestrel/copper intrauterine device (IUD) may also be an option. The progesterone-only pill, progesterone implant, combined contraceptive patches and vaginal ring are not recommended as they cannot be guaranteed to be effective.

For emergency contraception, a single dose of levonorgestrel, 3 mg, should be taken as soon as possible within 72 hours of unprotected intercourse. Ulipristal acetate is not recommended because of reduced efficacy; however, inserting a non-hormonal IUD within 5 days of intercourse is an alternative option.[1-3]

In general, OCPs do not reduce the efficacy of ASM. The exception is LTG, and women must be informed of this interaction. Any estrogen-based contraceptive can cause a significant reduction in plasma concentrations of LTG, resulting in loss of seizure control. LTG dose adjustment may be required when a woman starts taking these contraceptives. Progesterone-only contraceptives do not interact with LTG and can be used without restriction. Women with epilepsy taking other non-enzyme-inducing ASM (Table 8.2) should be informed that there is no known interaction with hormonal contraceptives. [1-3]

TABLE 8.1

Hormonal contraceptive advice for women with epilepsy taking enzyme-inducing ASM

Enzyme-inducing ASM	Recommended	Not recommended	Additional information
CBZ CEN ESL OXC PER (≥12 mg/day) PB PHT PRM RFN TPM (≥200 mg/day)	• Combined OCP must provide ≥50 µg/day of estrogen • If breakthrough bleeding with no other obvious cause, consider increasing to estrogen, 70 µg/day, and tricycling • Seek guidance on dosage of combined OCP from the SmPC and latest editions of national formularies • Use depot/subcutaneous progesterone and levonorgestrel IUDs **Emergency contraception** • Single-dose levonorgestrel, 3 mg, as soon as possible within 72 hours of unprotected intercourse • Do not use ulipristal acetate; insert non-hormonal IUD within 5 days of intercourse instead • Ensure type and dose of emergency contraception is in line with the SmPC and latest editions of national formularies	• Progesterone-only pill • Progesterone implant • Combined contraceptive patches • Vaginal ring	• Discuss additional barrier methods, alternative oral contraception or depot progestogen injections • Non-hormonal barrier methods are less effective than combined OCP; non-hormonal IUD may be contraceptive of choice • Risk of bone loss with depot/subcutaneous progesterone

Adapted from Shepley 2016.[3]

TABLE 8.2

Hormonal contraceptive advice for women with epilepsy taking non-enzyme-inducing ASM

Non-enzyme-inducing ASM	Recommendations
Acetazolamide	• As for women not taking an ASM
BRV	• Non-enzyme-inducing ASM do not alter the effectiveness of combined contraceptive patches, combined OCP, progesterone-only pill, progesterone implant, vaginal ring or emergency contraceptives
CLB	
Clonazepam	
ESM	
GBP	
LCM	**Emergency contraception**
LEV	• As for women not taking an ASM
PER (< 12 mg/day)	• Progestogen-only contraceptives can be used without restriction
PGB	
VPA	• LTG clearance is doubled by ethinyl estradiol/levonorgestrel, 30 μg/150 μg, threatening seizure control; an increased LTG dose may be required
TGB	
TPM (≥ 200 mg/day)	• Women should be made aware of signs and symptoms of LTG toxicity; the LTG dose should be reduced if these occur
VGB	
ZNS	• Desogestrel may increase LTG concentrations
LTG	
	Emergency contraception
	• As for women not taking an ASM

Adapted from Shepley 2016.[3]

Menstruation

Up to 40% of women find that their seizures worsen during their menstrual cycle, a phenomenon known as catamenial epilepsy. This exacerbation is thought to be a consequence of an imbalance between estrogen and progestogen concentrations. Hormonal preparations that induce amenorrhea can be successful in reducing catamenial epilepsy. Keeping a diary of menstrual cycles and seizure activity may help to determine when to optimize the use of an ASM such as intermittent CLB for the few days just before and shortly after the onset of menstruation.[4]

An observational cohort study comparing fertility in women with epilepsy who had no previous diagnosis of fertility-lowering disorders (such as polycystic ovaries) with fertility in control women without epilepsy, found that women with epilepsy had similar pregnancy rates and times to conception as the control women.[5] Some women with epilepsy taking VPA have a higher rate of menstrual dysfunction and increased risk of polycystic ovary syndrome,[6] which are reversible when VPA is discontinued. Some women with epilepsy may have difficulty conceiving, but they should not assume this is related to their ASM and should seek a second opinion from a gynecologist.

Pregnancy

Pregnant women with epilepsy are a high-risk group in outpatient and inpatient settings and their care ideally should be jointly managed by an epilepsy specialist and an obstetrician. Although most women with epilepsy (93%) have normal pregnancy outcomes,[7] epilepsy continues to be one of the main contributors to maternal mortality. The UK and Ireland Confidential Enquiries into Maternal Deaths and Morbidity 2016–2018 identified 22 maternal deaths during pregnancy and up to 6 weeks postpartum, representing a mortality rate of 0.91 per 100 000 maternities (95% CI 0.58, 1.38), more than double the rate of SUDEP identified in a previous report. The case histories of 19 women were examined closely in the report. Very few had documented advice before pregnancy, the majority had uncontrolled epilepsy, four were not taking ASM, eight were taking LTG (the plasma concentration of which can fall during pregnancy), and fewer than 50% had specialist review throughout pregnancy.[8]

Preconception. Girls and women with epilepsy should be offered effective contraception to avoid unplanned pregnancies. Those with uncontrolled seizures need to stabilize their epilepsy by optimizing their ASM, then plan their pregnancy, aiming for positive pregnancy outcomes. Although it would be ideal to withdraw ASM to minimize the risk of major congenital malformation (MCM) in the fetus, for many women this would result in recurrence or exacerbation of seizures that could be dangerous for both mother and fetus.[8] If the criteria for discontinuation are met, the ASM should be stopped over a suitable interval before conception. If the ASM cannot be withdrawn completely, it should be tapered to the minimum effective dose of, if possible, a single drug. All women on ASM should take supplemental folic acid, 4–5 mg daily, from at least 3 months before conception until birth to reduce the risk of neural tube defects.[9] Guidelines for managing epilepsy in women who are planning pregnancy are detailed in Table 8.3.

During pregnancy. Once pregnancy has been confirmed the woman needs to be referred to her usual epilepsy specialist, ideally within 2 weeks. Best practice guidelines[10] recommend that a woman's pregnancy be jointly managed by obstetric and epilepsy services. During pregnancy, metabolic processes change and close attention should be paid to ASM concentrations. Total serum concentrations of some drugs will fall, particularly those of PHT (Figure 8.1) and LTG. The implications for seizure control and frequency are difficult to predict.

A double-blind randomized trial (EMPiRE)[11] did not find monitoring serum ASM levels during pregnancy to be effective. However, the trial found that pregnant women cared for effectively by epilepsy and obstetric services working in partnership reported feeling educated and cared for. Women whose epilepsy is well controlled usually remain seizure free during pregnancy and delivery. Conversely, those who continue to report seizures before conception may have increased seizures during pregnancy.

Fetal health. The incidence of MCM in children born to women with epilepsy is approximately three times higher than in those born to women without epilepsy.[12] The risk increases disproportionately with the number of drugs being taken: it is approximately 3% for one drug (similar to background risk), 5% for two, 10% for three and over 20% in women taking more than three ASM (Figure 8.2). VPA is highly teratogenic and carries a 10% risk of MCM and 30–40% risk of neurodevelopmental, cognitive and behavioral disorders following in-utero exposure.[13] VPA should be avoided in pregnancy unless there are no other ASM options.

The teratogenic risk associated with CBZ, LTG and LEV is low. Studies have shown the MCM risk associated with in-utero exposure to be 2.6% with CBZ (95% CI 1.9, 3.5), 2.3% with LTG (95% CI 1.8, 3.1)[14]

TABLE 8.3

Guidelines for managing epilepsy in girls and women planning pregnancy

- Consultation with a healthcare professional with expertise in epilepsy management is essential
- Verbal and written information should be given, with the following advice
  - Most women with epilepsy have normal pregnancy outcomes
  - Do not suddenly stop taking your ASM if you realize you are pregnant
  - The risk of congenital abnormalities in the fetus depends on the type, number and dose of ASM
- If contemplating ASM withdrawal, a thorough discussion about the risks and benefits (including risk of SUDEP) before conception is essential
- Review ASM regimen before conception, aiming for monotherapy (if possible) with the lowest effective dose of ASM (consider splitting doses of ASM, e.g. from once daily to twice daily, or from twice daily to three times daily, to reduce individual dose)
  - Individuals taking VPA and ASM such as PHT, TPM and ZNS should be counseled about changing their medication before conception after a careful evaluation of the potential risks and benefits
  - Individuals taking VPA need to be informed about the possible adverse effects on long-term neurodevelopment following in-utero exposure
- Inform all girls and women with epilepsy, especially women experiencing seizures while asleep or uncontrolled seizures while awake and who are drug-resistant, about SUDEP and the risk of miscarriage
- Discuss available antenatal screening and the need for frequent ASM measurements during pregnancy and for at least 8 weeks after delivery
- Prescribe folic acid, 4–5 mg daily, at least 3 months before conception and continue until birth
- Advise about the need for strict ASM adherence and adequate sleep throughout pregnancy
- Document each of the above in the individual's medical record

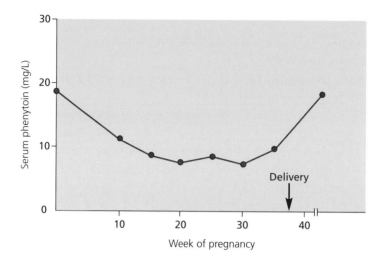

Figure 8.1 Serum PHT concentrations during pregnancy and delivery in a woman taking an established dose of 300 mg daily.

and 0.70% with LEV (95% CI 0.19, 2.51).[15] The risk of MCM associated with TPM was found to be higher in women taking more than 100 mg per day (5.16%; 95% Cl 1.94, 13.73).[16] ZNS was teratogenic in animal studies but there is limited information on MCM in human fetuses. As there is the possibility of an increased risk of MCM, women need to be carefully counseled about it.[17] There are insufficient data regarding the safety of other modern ASM.

After birth. The older enzyme-inducing ASM (CBZ, PHT, PB and PRM) can cause transient and reversible deficiencies in vitamin K1-dependent clotting factors in the neonate. The risk of intracerebral hemorrhage increases if the birth is traumatic. All babies at risk should receive 1 mg intramuscular vitamin K immediately after birth. There is insufficient evidence for routine maternal use of oral vitamin K.[1,2]

After delivery. All mothers taking ASM should be encouraged to breastfeed their babies and/or be supported to choose the feeding method that best suits mother and baby. The concentrations of PHT, CBZ and VPA in breast milk are low and not usually harmful. High doses of ASM, polytherapy and regimens that include PRM, LEV, GBP,

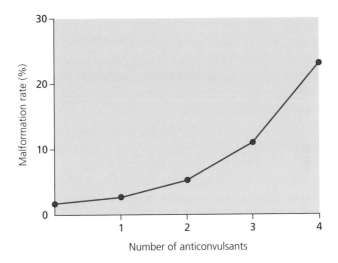

Figure 8.2 Relationship between number of antiepileptic drugs taken during the first trimester of pregnancy and the likelihood of fetal malformation. Data from Nakane Y et al. *Epilepsia* 1980;21:663–80.

LTG and TPM may cause sedation. If a baby is found to be drowsy or sedated, breastfeeding should be alternated with bottle feeding. If there is a change to the baby's behavior, feeding pattern and growth, breastfeeding should switch to bottle feeding entirely.[1,2]

Care of the infant. Women should be reassured that the risk to their baby from maternal seizures is usually low. Women with seizure types that involve loss of awareness and myoclonic jerks should consider their baby's safety especially when bathing, feeding and carrying. General advice includes never bathing the baby alone and sitting on soft floor furnishings when feeding.[1–3]

Contraception postpartum. Women with epilepsy need contraceptive advice after delivery to avoid an unplanned pregnancy. Progesterone-only oral contraceptives are usually the method of choice in breastfeeding women but are contraindicated for women with epilepsy taking hepatic enzyme-inducing ASM (see Table 8.1).[1,2] Alternative hormonal and non-hormonal contraceptives are options to consider.

Pregnancy registries. The European Registry of Antiepileptic Drugs and Pregnancy (eurapinternational.org) was launched in 1999. It is a consortium of independent research groups whose primary objective is to compare the risks of MCM associated with ASM use during pregnancy and share them in an international registry. A secondary objective is to evaluate specific patterns of fetal abnormalities, dose-effect relationships and other risk factors. Clinicians from 46 countries in Europe, Oceania, Asia, Latin America and Africa have contributed to the registry and more than 28 000 pregnancies had been registered by 2021.

The North American (Antiepileptic Drug) Pregnancy Registry was established in 1997 to help pregnant women determine prospectively the risk of MCM associated with ASM. Over 13 500 women had enrolled by February 2021.

The UK Epilepsy and Pregnancy register was established in 1996 for pregnant women in the UK. The main objective is to obtain and publish information on the frequency of malformations such as heart defects, spina bifida and cleft lip among infants whose mothers take one or more ASM. Women with epilepsy who become pregnant, either taking ASM or not, are eligible to register but must do so early in pregnancy and before the outcome is known.

Teenagers

The time leading up to and during the transition of teenagers with epilepsy from pediatric to adult healthcare services is particularly important. Joint care between clinicians caring for children with epilepsy and clinicians caring for adults with epilepsy in a transition clinic is recommended. Teenagers should be empowered to manage their own epilepsy and be given age-appropriate information on matters such as contraception, pregnancy, driving, employment, alcohol and other lifestyle choices, alongside support to help them live with epilepsy (see *Fast Facts: Epilepsy in Children and Adolescents* for more detailed information).[1,2]

Women and the menopause

All women with epilepsy entering menopause should receive individualized accurate advice and information about the interaction between hepatic enzyme-inducing ASM and hormone replacement therapy (HRT).[1] Estrogen in HRT formulations can reduce LTG concentrations significantly and dose adjustments are usually necessary. There is very little research evidence about the effect of menopause on epilepsy, although some women may experience an increase in seizures as a result of changing estrogen levels. Consideration needs to be given to bone health after menopause and vitamin D supplementation is recommended to improve bone density.[2]

Elderly patients

The number of elderly people being diagnosed with epilepsy is likely to rise further with aging populations. Elderly patients are more likely to have focal-onset seizures with or without bilateral tonic–clonic seizures, many of which arise from sleep. An underlying symptomatic etiology can be identified in a larger proportion of elderly people than in younger individuals. Stroke (ischemic or hemorrhagic) and other cerebrovascular diseases, such as cerebral vein and sinus thrombosis, or vascular malformations account for 30–50% of cases. Primary neurodegenerative disorders associated with cognitive impairment, such as Alzheimer's disease and dementia, account for 10–20%. Head trauma, often due to falls, accounts for 10–20% and brain tumors account for 10–30%.[18] New-onset idiopathic syndromes are rare.

The diagnosis of epilepsy can be challenging in older people and depends on a witnessed event. However, an assessment of the likelihood of seizures often has to be made on circumstantial evidence, as a proportion of older people live alone and/or have no bed partner to observe seizures from sleep. Focal impaired-awareness seizures, presenting as confusion, may be misdiagnosed as psychiatric symptoms. Postictal confusion can be prolonged in the elderly and may contribute to physical injury sustained during a seizure.

ASM is the mainstay of treatment and is effective in most patients. Complete seizure control can be expected in more than 70% of elderly patients. A subgroup, often with progressive neurodegenerative diseases such as Alzheimer's and dementia, will continue to have seizures despite all attempts at pharmacological prevention. Additional support may be required for these elderly patients; it is important to undertake memory and cognitive functioning assessments to identify need and the level of care required. Multidisciplinary services in the community setting must be utilized from diagnosis and provide rehabilitation and long-term management.

Elderly patients are particularly sensitive to the adverse effects of ASM, possibly because of age-related pharmacokinetic changes caused by the delay in gastric emptying, reduction in body fat and decreased hepatic metabolism and renal elimination. Low doses are generally recommended in the elderly to minimize adverse effects. The person with epilepsy, and often their spouse and children, must be convinced of the need for lifelong treatment. Sympathetic explanation and assured support will help an elderly person regain their self-confidence after epilepsy has been diagnosed and ASM established. The choice of drug depends on the side-effect and interaction profiles. Drugs with a high propensity for neurotoxicity should be avoided (see Table 4.2).

In people using multiple concomitant medications, drugs that do not produce pharmacokinetic interactions are the preferred choice (see Table 4.3). Few clinical trials of ASM have been performed specifically in the elderly. Double-blind trials support LTG over CBZ for the treatment of focal-onset seizures and bilateral tonic–clonic seizures (GTCS), primarily because it produces fewer neurotoxic side effects. LEV is a suitable alternative, but it should be used cautiously in elderly people with mental health problems as it is associated with an increased risk of worsening anxiety and depression despite being well tolerated in this population and implicated in fewer drug interactions than all other ASM.

Elderly people with epilepsy are also emotionally affected by social and physical restrictions to their lifestyle. The impact of driving restrictions affects them just as it does younger people. Falls and resulting injuries from seizures are more likely to occur in elderly people, causing those affected to lose confidence and independence.

People with intellectual and developmental disabilities

Epilepsy has a prevalence of 22.2% (95% CI 19.6, 25.1) in people with ID. Prevalence increases from 10% in people with mild ID to 30% in those with moderate, severe or profound ID.[19] Diagnosis relies heavily on an accurate description of events. In particular, focal-onset seizures can be mistaken for behaviors potentially associated with autism, and vice versa. Seizures in Rett syndrome can be particularly problematic to diagnose.

Some people with ID have difficulty tolerating investigations. However, every attempt should be made to offer the full range of diagnostic tests. Reasonable adjustments such as allowing more time to explain procedures and perform the studies or undertaking ambulatory EEG in the home environment, should be considered. Despite this, even specialist clinics report lower than expected use of diagnostic tests for people with ID.[20]

The types of seizures experienced by people with ID will vary according to the syndromic diagnosis. Some syndromes, such as DS and LGS, are heavily associated with ID, and the resultant seizures can be extremely difficult to treat. There is often a temptation to use high-dose polypharmacy to try to manage seizures, but this may be detrimental to overall quality of life. However, clinicians must resist any feelings of nihilism, and make every effort to reduce an individual's seizure burden. Often 'fresh eyes' on a case can transform lives.[21] It must also be remembered that epilepsy is one of the top causes of preventable mortality and hospitalization for people with ID.[22] There is certainly a role for VNS and dietary approaches for these people. Resective surgery should not be discounted on the grounds of ID.

The management of people with ID is complex and should be undertaken by a multidisciplinary team. The needs of this group of people were highlighted by an ILAE/International Bureau for Epilepsy-sponsored White Paper published in 2014.[23] This outlined four domains requiring concerted international action:
• the development of standards and initiatives to enhance diagnosis, investigative pathways and treatment
• guidelines for treatment, specifically best practice in the management of ASM
• standards for primary care, multidisciplinary teamwork and clinical consultations with an emphasis on enhancing communication and access to information
• the enhancement of links across different stakeholders, organizations and services.

A recent report outlined the components of a desirable epilepsy service for people with ID (Table 8.4).[21] It is unlikely that most

TABLE 8.4

Desirable components of an epilepsy service for people with ID

Medical services

- ID psychiatrist (or child and adolescent psychiatrist) with epilepsy interest and a neurologist with ID interest*

- Neurologist with ID interest

Clinics

- Dedicated joint epilepsy and ID clinics *

- Dedicated clinics for people with ID in a general neurology epilepsy setting, or epilepsy-dedicated clinic in an ID or child and adolescent mental health ID setting

- Adequate time to inquire into epilepsy issues in ID clinics

There are risks as well as benefits to creating separate clinics for people with ID and epilepsy. Delivery of standards of care in both epilepsy and ID needs to be assured.

It is also worth considering using video or teleconsultation to facilitate joint clinical participation of epilepsy and ID professionals.

Nursing service

- ID nurse with epilepsy interest*

- Epilepsy nurse with ID interest*

Multidisciplinary team

Consisting of occupational therapist, physiotherapist, psychologist, speech and language therapist, dietitian and social worker

- Dedicated team for epilepsy *

- ID-based with neurology access

Epilepsy surgery

- On site*

- Link to tertiary center

Pediatric-to-adult transition

- Joint clinic*

- Young people's epilepsy clinic

- ID or neurological clinic

- Agreed pathway

*Ideal service components.
Reproduced with permission from Shankar and Mitchell 2020.[21]

services for people with ID will have clinicians possessing an in-depth knowledge of neurology, while neurologists will not usually be well versed in the management of people with ID. The principal therefore is for collaborative working, as close cooperation between services can minimize shortfalls and optimize outcomes for people with epilepsy and ID. Such an integrated model is outlined in Figure 8.3.

Since 2016, the UK epilepsy and ID register, in collaboration with pan-European researchers, has compared the efficacy and tolerability of specific ASM in people with severe-to-profound ID, versus those with mild-to-moderate ID, versus those without ID. Several papers have now been published, with some differences noted. For example,

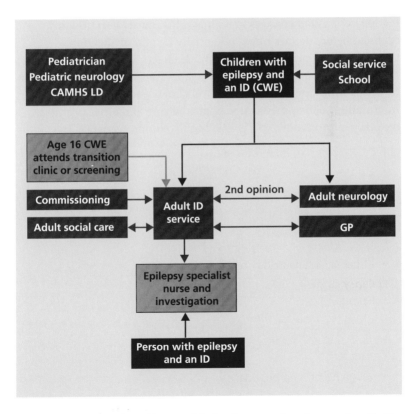

Figure 8.3 Integrated working model of epilepsy services for people with ID. Reproduced with permission from Shankar and Mitchell 2020.[21]

the tolerability of PER seems to be better for those with severe-to-profound ID than those with mild-to-moderate or no ID.[24]

While data are lacking, some general recommendations for the use of ASM in people with ID can now be made (Table 8.5). Important considerations are efficacy, which should primarily be based on seizure type, with particular care taken to avoid contraindicated drugs such as CBZ or PHT in patients experiencing absences, myoclonic jerks, tonic or atonic seizures as part of their syndromic presentation. Similarly, drugs with minimal cognitive and/or behavioral side effects are preferred. Diagnostic overshadowing is a serious consideration here, with behavioral changes often blamed on ASM by family or professional carers. Other reasons, both physical and environmental, for apparent mood changes in an individual must be thoroughly explored before deprescribing potentially helpful medication. Conversely, potentially serious ASM side effects can be overlooked, particularly when people with ID are supported at clinic appointments by people who do not know them well and do not bring vital information such as medication charts, seizure and other healthcare records. Unfortunately, this is an all-too-common scenario.

TABLE 8.5

Evidence and suitability of specific commonly used ASM in the ID population

Drug	ID-specific evidence	Type of evidence	Commentary	Level of evidence*	Suitability in ID**
LTG	Motte et al. 1997	LGS specific; RCT using placebo	Under powered, specific syndrome	I	**Recommendation** Should be considered as first-line treatment
	Buchanan 1995	n=34; majority showed >50% improvement	Under powered		**Pros** One of the most well-studied molecules in both general and ID populations
	Gidal et al. 2000	n=44; 45% showed >50% improvement; 20% showed worsening	Under powered		**Cons** Possible interactions; slow titration to dose
	McKee et al. 2006	n=22; subanalysis of a larger study	Under powered		

CONTINUED

TABLE 8.5 CONTINUED

Evidence and suitability of specific commonly used ASM in the ID population

Drug	ID-specific evidence	Type of evidence	Commentary	Level of evidence*	Suitability in ID**
VPA	Marson et al. 2007	Subanalysis of difficult-to-treat epilepsy	Multiple methodological issues	V	**Recommendation** Should be considered as first-line treatment; however, only to be used in exceptional circumstances if person with ID (usually borderline to mild ID) is a sexually active female of child-bearing age **Pros** First-line ASM with recognized suitable mood profile **Cons** Risk of polycystic ovarian syndrome **Other** One of the most used ASM in people with ID despite limited evidence in people with ID

LEV	Kelly et al. 2004	n=64; observational study of adjunct LEV; 38% seizure free	Improved seizure control in majority and carer satisfaction	III	**Recommendation** To be considered if benefits outweigh risks or as second-line treatment
	Brodtkorb et al. 2004	n=184 (56 with ID); equally effective	Study focus was on behavior (worse in ID)		**Pros** Does not interact with other commonly prescribed medication in people with ID; well studied in the general population and considered first-line medication **Cons** Needs more studies in ID; concerns about behavioral and mental side effects (though these may be more common in the general population than in people with ID due to titration differences)

CONTINUED

149

TABLE 8.5 CONTINUED

Evidence and suitability of specific commonly used ASM in the ID population

Drug	ID-specific evidence	Type of evidence	Commentary	Level of evidence*	Suitability in ID**
TPM	Kerr et al. 2005	RCT double blind to placebo n=57 divided 28/29, 32% or treatment group showed reduction in seizure frequency vs. 1% in placebo	No negative impact on behavior; Under power	I	**Recommendation** To be considered if benefits outweigh risks or as second-line treatment **Pros** Reasonable evidence in ID; no major interactions other than with oral contraceptives **Cons** The RCT found no effect on behavior, but real-world experience suggests it can affect mood and behavior; weight loss
GBP	Crawford et al. 2001	Add-on comparative open study with LTG; no difference found	Under powered; side effects of aggression	II	**Recommendation** To be considered if benefits outweigh risks or as second-line treatment **Other** No definitive details of efficacy or potential for harm

| PER | Shankar et al. 2017 | Retrospective case series; n=144 (general population 71, mild ID 48, moderate-to-profound ID 25) | >50% seizure improvement in 24% of those with mild ID, 26% of those with moderate-to-profound ID; safe in people with ID and better tolerated than in general population; mental health side effects | III | **Recommendation**
To be considered if benefits outweigh risks or as second-line treatment

Pros
Does not usually interact with other commonly prescribed medication in people with ID; well studied in the general population and people with ID in real-world studies; a viable alternative in treatment-resistant epilepsy

Cons
Concerns about behavioral and mental side effects |

CONTINUED

TABLE 8.5 CONTINUED

Evidence and suitability of specific commonly used ASM in the ID population

Drug	ID-specific evidence	Type of evidence	Commentary	Level of evidence*	Suitability in ID**
LCM	Flores et al. 2012	Real-world cohort; n=403 (18% with ID); no differences between ID and non-ID	Case selection	IV	**Recommendation** To be considered if benefits outweigh risks or as second-line treatment
					Pros Favorable side-effect profile
					Cons Needs more evidence

					Recommendation
CBZ	Kaski et al. 1991	Improved efficacy using slow-release preparation vs standard	No direct evidence of tolerability or efficacy	II (but unrelated)	To be considered if benefits outweigh risks or as second-line treatment **Pros** Long-standing ASM; recognized first-line treatment **Cons** No direct evidence of efficacy; multiple drug interactions with other commonly prescribed medication in people with ID (e.g. other ASM and psychotropics)
PHT	None	None	–	V	**Recommendation** Only use in exceptional circumstances; requires comprehensive discussion with patient of benefits and risks balanced against alternatives, efficacy and side effects **Cons** Multiple drug interactions; behavioral side effects; requires regular blood monitoring

CONTINUED

TABLE 8.5 CONTINUED

Evidence and suitability of specific commonly used ASM in the ID population

Drug	ID-specific evidence	Type of evidence	Commentary	Level of evidence*	Suitability in ID**
PB	None	None	–	V	**Recommendation** Only use in exceptional circumstances; requires comprehensive discussion with patient of benefits and risks balanced against alternatives, efficacy and side effects **Cons** Cognitive issues; multiple drug interactions; behavioral side effects; requires regular blood monitoring

Grading evidence: Ia, evidence from systematic reviews or meta-analysis of RCTs; Ib, evidence from at least one controlled study without randomization, and from at least one other type of quasi-experimental study; III, evidence from non-experimental descriptive studies, such as comparative studies, correlation studies and case-control studies; IV, evidence of post-study analysis of a section of the ID population following large sample studies.; V, evidence from expert committee reports or opinions and/or clinical experience of respected authorities (Adapted from Canadian Task Force on the Periodic Health Examination, 1979; Sackett, 1989).

RCT, randomized controlled trial.

Adapted from Royal College of Psychiatrists, 2017.[25]

Key points – specific populations

- Girls and women with epilepsy who are planning a pregnancy should be seen by healthcare professionals with expertise in epilepsy management and be provided with verbal and written information.
- Oral contraceptives containing at least 50 µg of estrogen should be used when co-administered with CBZ, ESL, FBM, OXC, PB, PHT, PRM and RFN, and TPM at doses over 200 mg daily, because these drugs induce metabolism of female sex hormones.
- The risk of MCM in babies exposed in utero seems to be greater with VPA than with other ASM.
- ASM is continued when necessary during pregnancy because seizures, especially convulsive seizures, are more harmful to the mother and fetus than the drugs themselves; however, treatment should be tapered to a minimally effective dose before pregnancy, if possible to a single ASM.
- A witness's account is particularly important for the correct diagnosis of epilepsy in the elderly, in whom the presentation of seizures is often subtle.
- Low doses of ASM are recommended in the elderly to minimize adverse effects, particularly neurotoxicity. Preferred choices include LTG and LEV.
- People with ID are more likely to develop epilepsy than the general population and epilepsy is one of the leading causes of mortality for people with ID.
- The treatment of people with ID and epilepsy can be complex and requires the skills of a multidisciplinary team to optimize management.

Key references

1. National Institute for Health and Care Excellence (NICE). *Epilepsies in Children, Young People and Adults. NICE guideline [NG217]*. National Institute for Health and Care Excellence, 2022. www.nice.org.uk/guidance/ng217, last accessed 6 June 2022.

2. Scottish Intercollegiate Guidelines Network. *Diagnosis and management of epilepsy in adults: a national clinical guideline*. Scottish Intercollegiate Guidelines Network, 2018. www.sign.ac.uk/media/1079/sign143_2018.pdf, last accessed 20 February 2022.

3. Shepley SA. Preconception to postpartum care: the need to maximise the safety of women with epilepsy. *Br J Neurosci Nurs* 2016;12:3.

4. Frank S, Tyson NA. A clinical approach to catamenial epilepsy: a review. *Perm J* 2020;24:1–3.

5. Pennell PB, French JA, Harden CL et al. Fertility and birth outcomes in women with epilepsy seeking pregnancy. *JAMA Neurol* 2018;75:962–9.

6. Markoula S, Siarava E, Keramida A et al. Reproductive health in patients with epilepsy. *Epilepsy Behav* 2020;113:107563.

7. Meador KJ, Baker GA, Browning N et al. Cognitive function at 3 years of age after fetal exposure to antiepileptic drugs. *N Engl J Med* 2009;360:1597–605.

8. Knight M, Bunch K, Tuffnell D et al. Saving Lives, Improving Mothers'Care: Lessons learned to inform maternity care from the UK and Ireland Confidential Enquiries into Maternal Deaths and Morbidity 2016–18. National Perinatal Epidemiology Unit, 2020. www.npeu.ox.ac.uk/assets/downloads/mbrrace-uk/reports/maternal-report-2020/MBRRACE-UK_Maternal_Report_Dec_2020_v10_ONLINE_VERSION_1404.pdf, last accessed 2 March 2021.

9. Kaplan YC, Koren G. Women using antiepileptic drugs: how much folic acid per day is sufficient? *Motherisk Int J* 2020;1:22.

10. Royal College of Obstetricians and Gynaecologists. Epilepsy in Pregnancy: Green-top Guidline No. 68. Royal College of Obstetricians and Gynaecologists, 2016. www.rcog.org.uk/globalassets/documents/guidelines/green-top-guidelines/gtg68_epilepsy.pdf, last accessed 2 March 2022.

11. Thangaratinam S, Marlin N, Newton S et al. AntiEpileptic drug monitoring in PREgnancy (EMPiRE): a double-blind randomised trial on effectiveness and acceptability of monitoring strategies. *Health Technol Assess* 2018;22:1–152.

12. Tomson T, Battino D, Bonizzoni E et al. Dose-dependent risk of malformations with antiepileptic drugs: an analysis of data from the EURAP epilepsy and pregnancy registry. *Lancet Neurol* 2011;10:609–17.

13. Medicines and Healthcare products Regulatory Agency. *Medicines related to valproate: risk of abnormal pregnancy outcomes.* GOV.UK, 2015. www.gov.uk/drug-safety-update/medicines-related-to-valproate-risk-of-abnormal-pregnancy-outcomes, last accessed 2 March 2022.

14. Campbell E, Kennedy F, Russell A et al. Malformation risks of antiepileptic drug monotherapies in pregnancy: updated results from the UK and Ireland epilepsy and pregnancy registers. *J Neurol Neurosurg Psychiatry* 2014;85:1029–34.

15. Mawhinney E, Craig J, Morrow J et al. Levetiracetam in pregnancy: results from the UK and Ireland epilepsy and pregnancy registers. *Neurology* 2013;80:400–5.

16. Hernandez-Diaz S, Huybrechts KF, Desai RJ et al. Topiramate use in pregnancy and the risk of oral clefts: a pregnancy cohort study. *Neurology* 2018;90:e342–51.

17. Medicines and Healthcare products Regulatory Agency. *Antiepileptic drugs: review of safety of use during pregnancy.* GOV.UK, 2021. www.gov.uk/government/publications/public-assesment-report-of-antiepileptic-drugs-review-of-safety-of-use-during-pregnancy/antiepileptic-drugs-review-of-safety-of-use-during-pregnancy, last accessed 2 March 2022.

18. Liu S, Yu W, Lu Y. The causes of new-onset epilepsy and seizures in the elderly. *Neuropsychiatr Dis Treat* 2016;12:1425–34.

19. Robertson J, Hatton C, Emerson E, Baines S. Prevalence of epilepsy among people with intellectual disabilities: a systematic review. *Seizure* 2015;29:46–62.

20. Tittensor PA, Rowe J, Youssef C et al. A structured, multi-disciplinary approach for the management of epilepsy for people with intellectual disabilities. *Epilepsy Professional* 2020;57:17–21. https://rwt.dspace-express.com/bitstream/handle/20.500.12687/312/Phil-Tittensor-A-Structured-Multi-Disciplinary-Approach-for-the-Management-of-Epilepsy.pdf?sequence=1, last accessed 2 March 2022.

21. Shankar R, Mitchell S. *Step Together. Integrating Care for People with Epilepsy and Learning Disability.* British Institute for Learning Disabilities, 2020. www.bild.org.uk/wp-content/uploads/2020/11/Step-Together-17-November-2020-Download-Link-.pdf, last accessed 2 March 2022.

22. University of Bristol. *Learning disability mortality review: action from learning report 2020/21.* NHS England, 2021. www.england.nhs.uk/wp-content/uploads/2021/06/LeDeR-Action-from-learning-report-202021.pdf, last accessed 2 March 2022.

23. Kerr M, Linehan C, Thompson R. et al. A White Paper on the medical and social needs of people with epilepsy and intellectual disability: the Task Force on Intellectual Disabilities and Epilepsy of the International League Against Epilepsy. *Epilepsia* 2014;55:1902–6.

24. Shankar R, Henley W, Wehner T et al. Perampanel in the general population and in people with intellectual disability: differing responses. *Seizure* 2017;49:30–5.

25. Royal College of Psychiatrists. *Prescribing anti-epileptic drugs for people with epilepsy and intellectual disability (CR206).* Royal College of Psychiatrists, 2017. www.rcpsych.ac.uk/improving-care/campaigning-for-better-mental-health-policy/college-reports/2017-college-reports/prescribing-anti-epileptic-drugs-for-people-with-epilepsy-and-intellectual-disability-cr206-oct-2017, last accessed 4 March 2022.

Further reading

National Institute for Health and Care Excellence (NICE). *CG110: Pregnancy and complex social factors: A model for service provision for pregnant women with complex social factors.* NICE, 2010. www.nice.org.uk/guidance/cg110, last accessed 9 March 2022.

Royal College of Pathologists. *Guideline G175: Deaths in patients with epilepsy including sudden deaths."* Royal College of Pathologists, 2019. Shankar R, Henley W, Boland C et al. Decreasing the risk of sudden unexpected death in epilepsy: structured communication of risk factors for premature mortality in people with epilepsy. *Eur J Neurol* 2018;25: 1121–7.

9 Comorbidities, quality of life and education

HEALTHCARE

Comorbidities

Comorbidity is very common in people with epilepsy, who often also experience psychiatric, neurological and cognitive conditions, either singularly or in combination. It is important to identify comorbid conditions at the time of diagnosis as they will affect treatment options, response to treatment, medical costs and quality of life.[1–3] A few studies have identified a bidirectional relationship between epilepsy and comorbid psychiatric and cognitive conditions, where one can affect the other and vice versa.[3,4]

Neuropsychiatric comorbidity. The risk of adults with epilepsy developing any psychiatric disorder is 2–5 times higher than the general population, with 1 in 3 adults with epilepsy receiving a psychiatric diagnosis at some time in their life.[2] The risk factors for psychiatric comorbidity may be biological, pharmacological and/or psychological.[3]

Depression is the most prevalent comorbid psychiatric condition in people with epilepsy, ranging from 20–55% in some studies and up to 70% in people with drug-resistant epilepsy.[5] A meta-analysis of risk factors for depression for people with epilepsy identified older age, female sex, low education level, unemployment, poor ASM adherence, polytherapy, stigma and anxiety as significant factors for increased risk, whereas marital status, economic level, age at seizure onset and seizure control did not increase the risk of depression.[6] A systematic review of neuroimaging studies of depression in adults with epilepsy found that depressive symptoms appeared to correlate highly with different patterns of brain changes specifically in temporal lobe epilepsy.[7]

Depression is underrecognized and, when diagnosed, often undertreated in people with epilepsy. Diagnosis may be further complicated if the individual minimizes their psychiatric symptoms, or if the clinician does not inquire about psychiatric symptoms or considers depression to be part of the normal adaptation to a diagnosis of epilepsy. Clinicians often treat depression inadequately because they are concerned that antidepressant therapy will increase seizure frequency.

The consequences of underdiagnosis and undertreatment can be fatal. A meta-analysis of studies conducted to quantify the relationship between epilepsy and suicide globally found 23.2% people with epilepsy had suicidal ideation (versus 3.1% in the general population), 7.4% had suicidal attempts and 0.5% completed suicidal death.[8] This has implications for ASM, as there is a class warning for increased suicide risk (see page 54).

Anxiety is the second most common comorbid psychiatric condition in people with epilepsy. One study identified a prevalence of anxiety disorders of 16.7% in people with epilepsy. Panic disorders were the most frequent manifestation of anxiety, observed in 13.5%.[9] Anxiety markedly compromises quality of life and psychosocial functioning. Ictal anxiety may be mistaken for a panic disorder. Patients experience anxiety most commonly interictally in the form of a generalized anxiety disorder. Severity of anxiety does not necessarily correlate with seizure frequency.

Treating neuropsychiatric comorbidity. Clinicians should evaluate people with epilepsy for anxiety and depression using simple screening instruments that are able to rapidly detect symptoms of these disorders in busy clinical settings.[10] If the patient is taking an ASM that is enhancing symptoms of anxiety and depression, consideration should be given to switching to another ASM that has a low risk of worsening psychiatric symptoms. The bidirectional relationship between anxiety/depression and epilepsy is complex, as anxiety and depression can increase seizure frequency and experiencing seizures can worsen anxiety and depression.[3]

A Cochrane review of the efficacy of antidepressants for people with epilepsy found limited evidence for their use. The trials assessed were small and larger, higher-quality trials are needed. Antidepressants such as venlafaxine and sertraline, together with CBT, may reduce depressive symptoms and improve the person's quality of life. None of the studies in this review identified antidepressants as a cause of deteriorating seizure control.[11] Therefore, promoting the use of complementary therapies and psychological interventions, especially CBT, alongside antidepressants, may improve both psychiatric comorbidity and quality of life of people with epilepsy.

Neurobehavioral comorbidity. Many neurobehavioral disorders affecting adults with epilepsy and ID originate in childhood. There is a spectrum of behavioral disorders that includes attention deficit hyperactivity disorder, autism spectrum disorder and developmental delays.[3] The choice of ASM is particularly important in this special population (see page 146 and Table 8.5).

Psychosis. A systematic review found that the prevalence of psychosis in epilepsy is estimated at 5.6% and is higher (7%) in temporal lobe epilepsy. The prevalence of interictal psychosis is 5.2% and postictal psychosis 2%.[12]

Ictal psychosis presents as hallucinations or delusions. Symptoms are usually self-limiting and can be mistaken for schizophrenia or mania, but unlike a primary psychiatric disorder are associated with a pattern of NCSE on EEG recording. Postictal psychosis generally begins years after the onset of epilepsy. The typical pattern is a cluster of focal impaired-awareness seizures, followed by a lucid postictal period. In turn, this lucid period is followed by affective symptoms together with grandiose and religious delusions, as well as focal auditory hallucinations. Patients with bilateral seizure foci, bilateral limbic lesions and clusters of focal impaired-awareness seizures are at particularly high risk.

Interictal psychosis also manifests as delusions and hallucinations, but disorganized behavior and thought disorders may also occur. Compared with patients with schizophrenia, patients with interictal psychosis have an absence of negative symptoms, a better premorbid state, less deterioration of personality and better response to pharmacotherapy.

Impaired cognitive comorbidity is also underrecognized and often untreated in adults with epilepsy. Research has shown that cognitive disturbances have affected some people with epilepsy before the onset of seizures and multiple causes, including pre-existing brain damage, seizures, interictal epileptic discharges, side effects of ASM and brain surgery, have been postulated. Comorbid cognitive impairments can have a negative impact on people with epilepsy and result in poor quality of life.[4]

The bidirectional relationship between cognitive impairment and epilepsy is also complex. Experiencing seizures can cause reversible cognitive impairment (as a result of ictal and postictal cognitive dysfunction) and interictal discharges negatively affect cognitive performance. However, cognitive and/or behavioral interventions have been shown to interrupt the start of a seizure.[13]

Cognitive impairments can cause people with epilepsy to become distressed especially when experiencing short-term memory loss, difficulty remembering faces and word finding. They need to be informed that cognitive impairments are common and that using external memory aids may be helpful. Neurological centers may be able to offer neuropsychological assessments to evaluate memory functioning. Complementary therapies and psychological interventions may help in reducing anxiety caused by cognitive impairment (see Chapter 6).

Quality of life

Receiving a diagnosis of epilepsy in adulthood can mean a great deal of lifestyle change. Restrictions on independence can be the most socially disabling, in particular the effects of epilepsy on employment, driving, life insurance and lifestyle. Accepting their diagnosis and adjusting their lifestyle (see Chapter 6) can enable people with epilepsy to live as normal a life as anybody else.

Employment is important for self-esteem and supporting an independent lifestyle. A diagnosis of epilepsy is more strongly linked with higher unemployment rates, job layoffs, being deemed unfit to work, feelings of shame for having epilepsy, lack of a life-partner and depression than other long-term conditions.[14] However, many people with epilepsy are able to work and carry out their duties safely and clinicians should encourage their patients to work whenever possible.

Resources are available for employers to help support people with epilepsy in the workplace. For example, the online 'Employers toolkit' (available at employers.epilepsy.org.uk) has risk assessment templates, seizure action plans and other resources covering matters such as first aid for seizures, safety and how to make reasonable adjustments in the workplace.

Driving is often viewed as essential to holding down a job and living independently. However, driving is a privilege. Applicants for a driver's license must meet the requirements of their state, province or country (see Useful resources, page 195). With reference to epilepsy, these requirements usually specify a seizure-free interval necessary for driving. Clinicians should be thoroughly familiar with the applicable laws where they practice and should clearly document their discussions with individuals with epilepsy. Clinicians should also remember that side effects of ASM, especially sedation, may interfere with a person's ability to safely operate a vehicle, and should advise them accordingly.

Life insurance. People with epilepsy may be unable to find affordable life insurance, particularly if applying for an individual policy. Most insurance companies ascribe a globally higher risk of mortality to people with seizures, irrespective of the applicant's frequency or severity of seizures. People with epilepsy should be encouraged to contact epilepsy charities as they work with many insurers and brokers to offer affordable insurance cover (see Useful resources, page 195).

Lifestyle modifications. Clinicians should counsel patients on lifestyle modifications that reduce the risk of provoking seizures and help maintain overall health without unduly limiting activities that bring enjoyment and fulfilment. Reducing or eliminating alcohol intake, engaging in stress-reducing behaviors, regular healthy eating and getting adequate sleep may help to reduce seizure frequency. Regular aerobic exercise, especially conducted in such a way that having a seizure would not pose a safety risk, is important for maintaining general health as well as bone health.

A systematic review of sport and physical activity found that people with epilepsy are physically less active and less fit than the general population. [15] However, most of the studies reviewed did not show evidence that physical activity increased seizure frequency.[15] Participation in low-risk sports such as dancing and golf should be encouraged, while individual risk assessments should be carried out for moderate-risk sports such as skiing/snow-boarding, swimming cycling and gymnastics.[15] With additional support and safety precautions people with epilepsy can continue to carry out many sporting and physical activities. Exceptions are extreme sports such as scuba diving and sky diving. While not banned by the relevant governing bodies, sports such as rock climbing and surfing carry significant risks, which should be carefully discussed.

Support groups. Epilepsy charities and organizations provide support for people with epilepsy in many ways, both practical and psychological (see Useful resources, page 195).

Education

Medication adherence. The importance of reminding people with epilepsy of the need to take their ASM as prescribed to reduce the risk of seizures cannot be underestimated; not doing so increases the risk of morbidity and mortality. A systematic review identified that ASM non-adherence in adults with epilepsy was associated with specific beliefs about taking medication, anxiety and depression, poor self-management, frequent daily dosing, poor relationships with clinicians and poor social support leading to poor seizure control and quality of life.[16] A Cochrane review found that behavioral interventions (intensive reminders) and mixed interventions (education and counseling) were positive strategies for improving adherence.[17] As cognitive impairments can result in people with epilepsy being forgetful, external memory aids, even something as simple as setting an alert on a cell phone, may be helpful.

Self-management tools. There is a wealth of easy-to-read information available in many formats from epilepsy charities and organizations that aims to help people with epilepsy, their families and clinicians learn about the condition and how to manage it. Resources include leaflets, fact sheets, first aid posters, seizure care plans and seizure diaries (see Useful resources, page 195).

Seizure care plans. People with epilepsy and their families should be empowered to take a central role in managing their condition. There are many examples of seizure care plans available for self-completion and/or to complete with clinicians. Developing care plans helps people with epilepsy make informed decisions about managing their condition, set goals and have at least an annual review to discuss issues that concern them.

Seizure diaries can be useful tools in clinical epilepsy reviews to monitor people's epilepsy, types of seizures and duration of seizures, as well as for identifying specific triggers, patterns and any medication change. This does depend on accurate recording and self-reporting has been found to be unreliable.[18] A review found that at least 50% of seizures were not remembered by patients during video-EEG monitoring.[19] Paper diaries are not always on hand after a seizure, therefore increasing the likelihood of forgetting, and they are often lost or not available during reviews. Online electronic diaries are potentially more useful.[19] Paper and electronic seizure diaries are freely available through epilepsy charities, and clinicians need to encourage people with epilepsy to complete them.

There are also apps available to help people with epilepsy monitor seizure frequency and type and reassess risk factors to determine whether risks are worsening, improving or staying the same. These encourage positive action and prompt a review of risks every 3 months.

Knowing the triggers for their seizures can help a person with epilepsy and their family learn how to modify their lifestyle to minimize the risk of occurrence. Some people may recognize a pattern (for example, in catamenial epilepsy when seizures occur around menstruation) or certain situations. Triggers vary from person to person, but the most common are forgetting to take an ASM (or deliberately not taking it), excess alcohol, lack of sleep/tiredness/sleep deprivation, stress/anxiety and illness (see Table 3.1 for more triggers).

Wearable devices such as wrist watches, armbands and smartphones allow detection of, and alert family members and carers to, motor seizure activity. However, more research is needed to determine the effectiveness and reliability of most of these devices. Wearable devices depend on capturing changes in movement and/or physiological signs and are not guaranteed to capture all seizure activity. No evidence has been found to determine whether non-EEG wearable devices are capable of detecting non-motor seizures,[18] nor has evidence been found that these wearable devices can prevent SUDEP.[20]

Two non-invasive wearable devices to detect tonic–clonic seizures in epilepsy have been approved by the US Food and Drug Administration and CE marked by the European Union. The 'Empatica Embrace' smartwatch measures a person's movement (accelerometry) and electrodermal activity. It maintains a Bluetooth link to a smartphone and sends an alert to a nominated emergency contact via cloud servers. 'Brain Sentinel' consists of an upper-arm strap with an adhesive patch designed to capture electromyography changes.[18] Other wrist-worn sensors are available to detect tonic–clonic seizures and information about these can be found on epilepsy charities' websites. However, in all cases there are cost and subscription charges to consider.

Other wearable devices include fall alarms and alarms that people can carry on their person and activate when they need help. The use of wearable devices may improve the recording of seizures and response to ASM. It is very important that the person with epilepsy and their family discuss the benefits and risks of wearable devices with their epilepsy team.

Other alarms and sensors that are not wearable, but are equally important, include epilepsy bed sensors, which can raise the alarm when people have tonic–clonic seizures while asleep, and seizure-alert dogs.

Identification. Medical identification cards and/or medical jewelry are very useful for people with epilepsy to carry on their person in the event of a seizure while away from home. Vital information should include their name, date of birth, address, that they have epilepsy, type of seizures, medication, allergies, first aid information and emergency contact numbers.

Key points – comorbidities, quality of life and education

- Depression and anxiety are common in people with epilepsy and have a significantly negative impact on quality of life.
- The potential benefit of treating depression and anxiety pharmacologically outweighs the risk of increased seizures.
- People with epilepsy should be encouraged to work whenever possible, and resources are available for employers to help them support people with epilepsy in the workplace.
- Legal restrictions on driving for people with epilepsy vary; clinicians should be aware of the relevant laws in their place of practice and must clearly document their discussion with individuals with epilepsy.
- People with epilepsy should be counseled on lifestyle modifications that reduce the risk of provoking seizures without unduly limiting activities.
- People with epilepsy should be empowered and given tools for shared decision-making to self-manage their condition.

Key references

1. Mula M. The comorbidities of epilepsy explained. *Expert Rev Neurother* 2020;20:1207–9.
2. Mula M, Kanner AM, Jetté N, Sander JW. Psychiatric comorbidities in people with epilepsy. *Neurol Clin Pract* 2021;11:e112–20.
3. Srinivas HV, Shah U. Comorbidities of epilepsy *Neurol India* 2017;65:S18–S24.
4. Kanner AM, Helmstaedter C, Sadat-Hossieny Z, Meador K. Cognitive disorders in epilepsy I: clinical experience, real-world evidence and recommendations. *Seizure* 2020;83:216–22.
5. Strober LB, Chapin J, Spirou A et al. Assessment of depression in epilepsy: the utility of common and disease-specific self-report depression measures. *Clin Neuropsychol* 2018;32:681–99.

6. Yang Y, Yang M, Shi Q et al. Risk factors for depression in patients with epilepsy: a meta-analysis. *Epilepsy Behav* 2020;106:107030.

7. Elkommos S, Mula M. A systematic review of neuroimaging studies of depression in adults with epilepsy. *Epilepsy Behav* 2021;115:107695.

8. Abraham N, Buvanaswari P, Rathakrishnan R et al. A meta-analysis of the rates of suicide ideation, attempts and deaths in people with epilepsy. *Int J Environ Res Public Health* 2019;16:1451.

9. Wiglusz MS, Landowski J, Cubala WJ. Prevalence of anxiety disorders in epilepsy. *Epilepsy Behav* 2018;79:1–3.

10. Kwon O-Y, Park S-P. Depression and anxiety in people with epilepsy. *J Clin Neurol* 2014;10:175–88.

11. Maguire MJ, Marson AG, Nevitt SJ. Antidepressants for people with epilepsy and depression. *Cochrane Database Syst Rev.* 2021;4:CD010682.

12. Clancy MJ, Clarke MC, Connor DJ et al. The prevalence of psychosis in epilepsy; a systematic review and meta-analysis. *BMC Psychiatry* 2014;14:75.

13. Helmstaedter C, Witt J-A. Epilepsy and cognition– a bidirectional relationship? *Seizure* 2017;49:83–9.

14. de Souza JL, Faiola AS, Miziara CSMG, de Manreza MLG. The perceived social stigma of people with epilepsy with regard to questions of employability. *Neurol Res Int* 2018;2018:4140508.

15. van den Bongard F, Hamer HM, Sassen R, Reinsberger C. Sport and physical activity in epilepsy. *Dtsch Arztebl Int* 2020;117:1–6.

16. O'Rourke G, O'Brien JJ. Identifying the barriers to antiepileptic drug adherence among adults with epilepsy. *Seizure* 2017;45:160–8.

17. Al-Aqeel S, Gershuni O, Al-Sabhan J, Hiligsmann M. Strategies for improving adherence to antiepileptic drug treatment in people with epilepsy. *Cochrane Database Syst Rev* 2020;10:CD008312.

18. Brinkmann BH, Karoly PJ, Nurse ES et al. Seizure diaries and forecasting with wearables: epilepsy monitoring outside the clinic. *Front Neurol* 2021; 12:690404.

19. Fisher RS, Blum DE, DiVentura B et al. Seizure diaries for clinical research and practice: limitations and future prospects. *Epilepsy Behav* 2012;24:304–10.

20. Jory C, Shankar R, Coker D et al. Safe and sound? A systematic literature review of seizure detection methods for personal use. *Seizure* 2016;36:4–15.

10 Psychogenic non-epileptic seizures

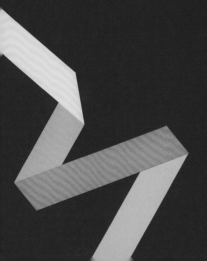

HEALTHCARE

PNES, also termed dissociative seizures, non-epileptic attack disorder, functional seizures and commonly, though unhelpfully, 'pseudoseizures', undoubtedly present the most challenging differential diagnosis for the epilepsy clinician. PNES were described as long ago as 1878 by the French neurologist Charcot, who used the term 'hystero-epilepsy'. He noticed that when people diagnosed with neurosis were placed on the same ward as people with epilepsy, they acquired symptoms resembling seizures.

Clinicians today often find it challenging to manage people with PNES.[1] Nevertheless, by approaching the diagnosis and subsequent management in a logical, stepwise manner, and working in partnership with the affected individual, the stereotype of poor prognosis can, for some people, be broken.

Epidemiology, pathophysiology and etiology

The overall incidence of PNES is thought to be 2–33 cases per 100000 people,[2] though this may be an underestimate, particularly following the civil restrictions that were imposed to counter the COVID-19 pandemic; anectodal evidence suggests a large increase in cases during this period. About 1 in 5 people presenting to a first seizure clinic will have PNES: 22% of people with PNES will also have epilepsy, while 16% of people with epilepsy will also have PNES.[3] Women are more likely to experience PNES than men, though estimates of the ratio vary.

Seizures most commonly begin in early adulthood, but they can present in children as young as 5 years old, or conversely in older people, often following life-changing physical events such as stroke. The diagnosis of PNES becomes even more challenging in the presence of such pathology, which also places the individual at higher risk of developing epilepsy. PNES are often frequent and prolonged, particularly soon after diagnosis, with a corresponding burden on health resources. It has been estimated that as many as 50% of people attending emergency departments with apparent SE are actually having prolonged PNES.

People with pre-existing psychological/psychiatric diagnoses, epilepsy, head injury and other brain pathology are at higher risk of developing PNES. These conditions can be thought of as the etiology of PNES, rather than the mechanism. The mechanism of PNES has been discussed in a theory that considers its heterogeneous nature and builds on an integrated model of other medically unexplained symptoms.[4]

The term PNES has largely been used by neurologists to denote the distinction between seizures caused by epilepsy and those that are medically unexplained. In many cases, an individual's attacks can be explained by another diagnosis, such as anxiety disorders, post-traumatic stress disorder, dissociative identity disorder, depersonalization disorder, factitious disorder or challenging behavior in the context of ID. According to integrated theory, placing PNES within the overall framework of a functional neurological disorder can be incorrect for a minority of people, though the vast majority fulfil the diagnostic criteria. Rather, the preconscious activation of a rogue mental representation by internal or external triggers appears to be common to all PNES, except those associated with factitious disorder. This is termed the 'seizure scaffold' (Figure 10.1). Rogue representations consist of cognitive, emotional or behavioral action programs that combine elements of inherent schemata, such as how to respond to fear, with the results of learning and experience in multiple situations.

What are schemata?

Patterns of thought or behavior that organize categories of information and the relationships among them. They can be described as a mental structure of preconceived ideas, a framework representing some aspect of the world or a system of organizing and perceiving new information.[5]

Activation of the seizure scaffold may or may not be associated with hyper- and hypoarousal (arousal levels not appropriate to the individual's current environment and internal state) and emotional or cognitive processing, accounting for the wide range of presentations of PNES.[4] Although abnormal arousal frequently occur in PNES, possibly giving rise to high-level processing dysfunction, it is not an essential aspect of the PNES generation process. For example, strong activation of the seizure scaffold in the presence of an inhibitory processing dysfunction may be sufficient to trigger an attack even in the absence of heightened arousal. Figure 10.1 focuses on how, rather than why, PNES arise. Recognized risk factors for PNES, such as a history of trauma, emotional dysregulation, alexithymia, psychopathology and heightened suggestibility, will confer vulnerability to the processes depicted, but are neither necessary nor sufficient to activate them.

Diagnosis

Misdiagnosis of PNES is common. Non-specialist misdiagnosis rates may approach 40%, while in neurology centers it is probably 10–20%. Even in tertiary epilepsy services a misdiagnosis rate of 5% is thought likely. The rule of two can be helpful: at least two normal EEGs, with at least two seizures per week and resistance to two ASM gives an 85% positive predictive value for PNES.[6]

PNES can be subclassified into several distinct seizure types, which fall into two broad categories:

- slumping attacks where the person lies motionless
- motor attacks, which manifest in different ways, though most involve trembling or shaking movements.

When taking a history, clinicians should examine the language used to describe the seizures. People with epilepsy tend to try to carefully describe the physical event, whereas people with PNES tend to describe the consequences of the seizure.[7]

The duration of PNES is often much longer than for epileptic seizures and seizures can also be serial, with or without full awareness returning between attacks. Similarly, recovery phases can be very different from those expected in epilepsy. Typically, the person may become orientated and coherent very quickly, though they may be tired for a prolonged period. Conversely, some people recover much more slowly from PNES than would be expected in epilepsy. It is very important to establish timeframes for each section of the event, particularly the postictal phase.

Witnesses to the attack should be asked about the individual's eyes: were they open, closed or rapidly blinking and, if opened by someone else, did they close as soon as the eyelid was released? Epileptic

Figure 10.1 Hypothesized sequence of events in PNES. Essential components of the process are represented in the dashed area. Reproduced from Brown and Reuber 2016, with permission of Elsevier.[4]

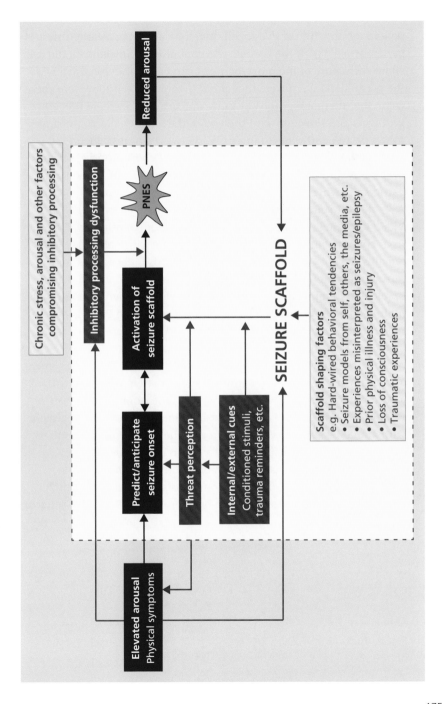

seizures occur with the eyes open, therefore anything different should be a clear red flag. If the episode was convulsive, clinicians should ask about the nature of the movements (it can be helpful to mime): was the person jerking, or were they more tremulous, as if they were very cold? Did the shaking stop abruptly (unlike a GTCS, where the jerks get bigger and slower toward the end of the seizure), did it stop and restart or wax and wane in intensity? SE, with repeated seizures, is unusual in people with established epilepsy. Reports of serial seizures over many minutes, or occasionally hours, should also be red flags, particularly when this is the habitual pattern.

Table 10.1 summarizes clinical signs favoring epilepsy or PNES. Video recordings can be extremely helpful in differentiating PNES from epilepsy but recording a habitual episode with video EEG remains the gold-standard diagnostic tool. This is dependent on the seizures being relatively frequent and the person accepting a period of telemetry; in practice, the scope for conclusive diagnostic testing is limited. Therefore, the level of diagnostic certainty in PNES is heavily reliant on the quality of witness history and the experience of the clinician (Table 10.2).

An uncertain diagnosis has major implications for the management and treatment of PNES as diagnostic doubt is often associated with a poor prognosis.[6] However, the length of time from the onset of symptoms to diagnosis is often measured in years. Initially, treatment with an ASM can improve PNES (though they rarely stop altogether), probably because of the placebo effect. This can perpetuate the misdiagnosis. The correct diagnosis often only emerges after the person has tried several drugs without consistent benefit, at which point they are reinvestigated, often by a tertiary-level epilepsy service.

TABLE 10.1

Differentiating epileptic seizures from PNES

Sign	Diagnostic level
Signs favoring PNES	
Long duration	Good
Fluctuating course	Good
Asynchronous movements	Good (frontal lobe focal seizures excluded)
Pelvic thrusting	Good (frontal lobe focal seizures excluded)
Side-to-side head or body movement	Good (convulsive events only)
Closed eyes	Good
Ictal crying	Good
Memory recall	Good
Signs favoring epileptic seizures	
Occurrence from EEG-confirmed sleep	Good
Postictal confusion	Good
Stertorous breathing	Good (convulsive events only)
Other signs	
Gradual onset	Insufficient
Non-stereotyped events	Insufficient
Flailing or thrashing movements	Insufficient
Opisthotonos or 'arc de cercle'	Insufficient
Tongue biting	Insufficient
Urinary incontinence	Insufficient

Adapted from La France et al. 2013.[6]

TABLE 10.2

Diagnostic levels of certainty for PNES

Diagnostic level	History	Witnessed event	EEG
Possible	+	By witness or self-report/description	No epileptiform activity in routine or sleep-deprived interictal EEG
Probable	+	By clinician reviewing video recording or witnessing in person, showing semiology typical of PNES	No epileptiform activity in routine or sleep-deprived interictal EEG
Clinically established	+	By clinician experienced in diagnosis of seizure disorders (on video or in person), showing semiology typical of PNES, while not on EEG	No epileptiform activity in routine or ambulatory ictal EEG during a typical ictus/event in which the semiology would make ictal epileptiform EEG activity expected during equivalent epileptic seizures
Documented	+	By clinician experienced in diagnosis of seizure disorders, showing semiology typical of PNES, while on video EEG	No epileptiform activity immediately before, during or after ictus captured on ictal video EEG with typical PNES semiology

+, history characteristics consistent with PNES.
Adapted from La France et al. 2013.[6]

Management and treatment

The management of PNES following diagnosis is often lacking.
A structured plan involving a multidisciplinary team and a named, primary point of contact for the individual (an epilepsy specialist nurse, neurologist, neuropsychiatrist or psychiatric nurse) would undoubtedly improve outcomes. A stepwise, holistic approach, recognizing the patient as an individual and accepting that no single treatment will work for everyone, should be the overarching principle of management.

Explaining PNES. It is vital that the diagnosing clinician takes time to clearly explain the condition (Table 10.3). This may need a much longer appointment than would be necessary in epilepsy. A clear explanation, particularly when the diagnosis has been made quickly, and the person has ongoing support, can render some people with

TABLE 10.3

Strategies used in communicating a diagnosis of PNES

Most useful concepts	Example language
Explain what PNES **is not** (i.e. epilepsy)	Good news, the seizures are not caused by epilepsy and therefore you don't need to take an ASM. The seizures are less dangerous (but acknowledge that it is still possible for them to cause injury).
Reassure that the seizures are real	These seizures happen at a subconscious level. You are not crazy. The seizures can be frightening or disabling and sometimes cause injury. You are not putting them on.
Give a name to the condition	These seizures have many different names, we prefer 'psychogenic non-epileptic seizures' or PNES, 'non-epileptic attack disorder', or 'dissociative' or 'functional' seizures, but you might hear terms like 'pseudoseizures', which many people with this condition do not like.
PNES is common	We see lots of people with these kinds of seizures. There are support groups, many of which are online via social media (signpost).
What PNES are	Seizures can be related to stress, emotion, difficult thoughts and memories. It's possible to get into a vicious cycle where there is worry or stress leading to more seizures, which leads to more stress. It can be hard to pinpoint triggers. Some people have a history of psychological trauma or abuse, but this isn't always the case (patients will often read about this, so it's almost always better to bring it up during the consultation).

CONTINUED

TABLE 10.3 CONTINUED

Strategies used in communicating a diagnosis of PNES

Other areas to discuss	Advice to give
Withdrawal of ASM (if prescribed)	This should be done gradually (the precise timing is based on the confidence of the individual).
Reassurance of support	Neurological follow-up will continue (ensure the person knows who to contact for advice between appointments). Psychology/psychiatry referral can be helpful.
Treatment	Seizures sometimes stop after a clear explanation. When they do not, psychological treatments are helpful (discuss what is available in your area and describe basic concepts of interventions like CBT).

Adapted from La France et al. 2013.[8]

PNES seizure free without more intensive treatment. Studies have suggested the most important concepts to cover in this early period (see Table 10.3).[8]

Pharmacological treatment. There is no specific medication for PNES. However, if the person is clinically depressed, then an antidepressant, typically a selective serotonin-reuptake inhibitor, can be helpful. Similarly, anxiolytics can sometimes be useful, but only if there is a clear diagnosis. Other pharmacological treatment should depend on physical diagnoses that may be having an effect on seizures. For example, a coexisting headache or migraine can worsen PNES, so effective headache management should be a priority in that situation. Pain is often a trigger for PNES, and fibromyalgia is a common comorbidity.

Psychological treatment. There is no single psychological treatment that will work for everyone with PNES. CBT is the approach with the most evidence, though a recent large multicenter trial (CODES) failed to demonstrate an overall reduction in seizures.[9] Secondary outcome measures showed significant improvements in overall health, and the principle of seeing seizures as a symptom of another underlying problem is a key concept in successful management.

Direct intervention aimed at aborting seizures can also be effective. Grounding techniques can be extremely useful if the person has a seizure warning. People can learn to modify their lifestyle in response to seizure triggers, in the same way that life hygiene principles can be useful in epilepsy (see Chapter 9). However, care needs to be taken to limit avoidance behavior, which can have a significant detrimental effect, causing social isolation and worsening seizures.

ACT has been studied in epilepsy. While there is currently no evidence in terms of large-scale trials for the use of this technique in PNES, the principles underpinning ACT, particularly mindfulness, can be hugely beneficial. Explaining the principle of treating the individual and their underlying diagnosis rather than purely counting seizures is a very helpful approach.

Other approaches. Several studies have suggested that relaxation techniques can be helpful in treating epileptic seizures, and it's possible they could also be useful in PNES. Aromatherapy, with or without hypnosis, may have a place here (see Chapter 9). Self-help techniques are described in detail at www.nonepilepticattacks.info. Brief, manualized, psychoeducational interventions delivered by non-psychologists can prove helpful,[10] though the data are mixed. Small case studies have reported improvements in PNES with eye movement desensitization and reprocessing. Group therapy and family therapy can be helpful for some people, as can anger and anxiety management courses.

Key points – psychogenic non-epileptic seizures

- PNES is the most challenging differential diagnosis for clinicians evaluating adults with suspected epilepsy; the term is used to denote the distinction between epileptic seizures and medically unexplained seizures.
- Two normal EEGs plus at least two seizures per week and resistance to two ASM give an 85% positive predictive value for PNES.
- PNES fall into the broad categories of slumping attacks and motor attacks.
- The level of diagnostic certainty in PNES depends heavily on the quality of witness history and clinician experience.
- A clear explanation of PNES following a rapid diagnosis, and with ongoing support, can lead to some people becoming seizure free without more intensive treatment.
- Pharmacological treatment of PNES focuses on comorbidities such as depression, anxiety, headache/migraine and pain.

References

1. Reuber M, Rawlins GH, Schachter SC, eds. *Non-Epileptic Seizures In Our Experience. Accounts of Healthcare Professionals.* Oxford University Press, 2020.
2. Kanemoto K, LaFrance Jr WC, Duncan R et al. PNES around the world: where we are now and how we can close the diagnosis and treatment gaps – an ILAE PNES Task Force report. *Epilepsia Open* 2017;2:307–16.
3. Kutlubaev MA, Xu Y, Hackett ML, Stone J. Dual diagnosis of epilepsy and psychogenic nonepileptic seizures: systematic review and meta-analysis of frequency, correlates, and outcomes. *Epilepsy Behav* 2018;89:70–8.
4. Brown RJ, Reuber M. Towards an integrative theory of psychogenic non-epileptic seizures (PNES). *Clin Psychol Rev* 2016;47:55–70.

5. Roesler C. *C. G. Jung's Archetype Concept. Theory, Research and Applications*. Taylor & Francis, 2021.

6. LaFrance Jr WC, Baker GA, Duncan R et al. Minimum requirements for the diagnosis of psychogenic nonepileptic seizures: a staged approach: a report from the International League Against Epilepsy Nonepileptic Seizures Task Force. *Epilepsia* 2013;54:2005–8.

7. Plug L, Sharrack B, Reuber M. Conversation analysis can help to distinguish between epilepsy and non-epileptic seizure disorders: a case comparison. *Seizure* 2009;18:43–50.

8. LaFrance Jr WC, Reuber M, Goldstein LH. Management of psychogenic nonepileptic seizures. *Epilepsia* 2013;54:53–67.

9. Goldstein LH, Robinson EJ, Mellors JDC et al. Cognitive behavioural therapy for adults with dissociative seizures (CODES): a pragmatic, multicentre, randomised controlled trial. *Lancet Psychiatry* 2020;7:491–505.

10. Mayor R, Brown RJ, Cock H et al. A feasibility study of a brief psycho-educational intervention for psychogenic nonepileptic seizures. *Seizure* 2013;22:760–5.

Neurology and Neuroscience

11 Research directions

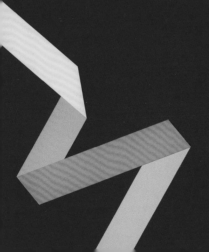

HEALTHCARE

Improving comparative datasets

One of the difficulties when researching long-term conditions is having sufficient data to be confident about the findings. Large research trials are expensive and a meta-analysis of several studies can be helpful. Unfortunately, because those disparate trials may have different methodologies, direct comparisons can be difficult. An international collaboration is under way to develop a core set of outcomes for epilepsy trials.[1] This should make it easier to compare data from different studies addressing the same question, thus allowing more data to be used in meta-analyses and providing more robust conclusions.

Artificial intelligence

AI has been used in several healthcare settings, most notably surgery, and computer-generated mathematical models are now being trialed in epilepsy. For example, algorithms to determine the risk of seizures from apparently normal brain data[2] and computer models that guide strategies for surgery[3] now offer a digital means of enhancing epilepsy diagnosis and care. Furthermore, improvements in wearable technology are enhancing care for people with epilepsy within the comfort of their own homes. These include devices that can detect absence seizures[4] and tonic–clonic seizures,[5] and technologies that enable long-term monitoring of EEG, such as UNEEG subscalp electrodes[6] or the ByteFlies sensor dot.[7] Seizures that occur during sleep can now be distinguished from other sleep phenomena using a computer algorithm to analyze video data. The Nelli system[8] has a high correlation with video telemetry but monitoring happens in the person's home without the need for electrodes. This is particularly helpful when assessing people with ID who may not be able to tolerate long-term (or any) EEG.

There is growing recognition that epilepsy, while sometimes a standalone condition, also has common comorbidities. The Multidisciplinary Expert System for the Assessment and Management of Complex Brain Disorders (MES-CoBraD)[9] is an attempt to develop a multidisciplinary diagnostic protocol, employing AI and machine learning techniques for neurocognitive disorders (dementia), sleep disorders and seizure disorders (epilepsy). It treats the three both individually and in any combination as a complex chronic condition to be investigated and treated in a multidisciplinary multidimensional manner.

Patient-centered research

In recent years, there has been increasing recognition that patients need to be leading players in the development of research questions. This means involving patients at every stage of the research process and ensuring that people living with epilepsy and their families and carers have a say in what is investigated. Effective and meaningful patient and public involvement (PPI) in health research has been shown to deliver benefits to research in terms of the relevance of the work and the efficacy of its delivery.[10] PPI also increases the democracy of the process by giving a 'voice' to those involved.[11] It provides transparency and accountability to funding decisions by ensuring organizations fund the research that matters most to those affected.

The benefits of PPI have been reflected in improvements in the relationships of people with epilepsy with those around them, as well as their employment, finances, health status, wellbeing and societal positions in terms of greater inclusion and equality. In Canada[12] and the UK,[13] epilepsy priority setting partnerships (PSPs) have been organized as a collaboration between the entire epilepsy community. National surveys have been conducted in both countries to collate the views of people living with epilepsy, their families, friends and carers, those bereaved by epilepsy, healthcare professionals and epilepsy charities. The information from these surveys will help to identify and prioritize areas of healthcare that can be improved by research and result in higher-quality studies and increased investment. In parallel with the PSPs, large numbers of people with epilepsy who want to be involved in research have joined groups such as Epilepsy Research UK's Shape Epilepsy Research Network, enabling them to influence epilepsy research and work with researchers to ensure their priorities are considered throughout the process.[14]

Preliminary analysis of the UK PSP suggests that the results are similar to those found in the Canadian PSP in 2021 (Table 11.1). Funding organizations are already beginning to use surveys like this to inform research grants.

TABLE 11.1

Top ten unanswered research questions from the Canadian Priority Setting Partnership (PSP)[12]

Priority	Question
1	Can genetic markers be used to diagnose and treat epilepsy and seizure disorders?
2	What are the impacts of long-term use of ASM, the causes of the side effects of these treatments and how can we prevent the side effects?
3	What are the long-term impacts of seizures on the person's brain, and overall health and development?
4	How can the risk of SUDEP be reduced in people with epilepsy?
5	What is the most effective testing protocol for determining causes of seizures and/or a diagnosis of epilepsy or other seizure disorders and to reduce time to diagnosis?
6	What are the brain changes, on a cellular level, that lead to seizure development?
7	How effective is surgical treatment for adults and children who experience seizures/epilepsy?
8	What causes memory problems associated with seizures? Can these memory problems improve over time and what are the best treatment options for memory loss in people who experience seizures?
9	Aside from ASM and some brain lesions, what causes behavioral changes in people who experience seizures? What is the best way to treat behavioral issues?
10	What is the efficacy (i.e. the effectiveness of reducing seizures) of adding a second ASM compared with changing to a different ASM? How can we determine which combinations of ASM are effective?

Big data research

Bringing together data on vast numbers of people with epilepsy and using new and emerging technologies to analyze these data, may provide new insights on epilepsy and accelerate innovations in research and future management of the condition.[15] Mathematical modeling can help to assess when and why epilepsy treatment fails to work. Data recordings from people with juvenile absence epilepsy and other GGE who are taking new ASM, and from people with focal epilepsy who have undergone surgery, are being analyzed for hidden features that may indicate why certain people continue having seizures while others become seizure free.[16] It is hoped that within the next 5–10 years this will contribute to the development of robust prognostic markers to help inform patient management and significantly improve self-management of seizures.

Understanding SUDEP

Research to understand why SUDEP happens, and who is most at risk, may help inform interventions to prevent epilepsy-related deaths and, ultimately, save lives. In some people with epilepsy, the respiratory and cardiovascular systems do not work optimally, especially during sleep. To better understand the cause of SUDEP, sophisticated brain network analysis is being applied to MRI data and EEG recordings from research centers around the world to study how connections between the brain regions that regulate heartbeat and breathing are altered in patients when they are awake and when they are asleep.[17] The brain connectivity in people who later died of SUDEP is being compared with that of living people during sleep and waking. This research will help to uncover why SUDEP frequently happens during sleep and will provide a better understanding of which brain regions and networks are affected in people who have subsequently died of SUDEP. It may suggest ways to identify people at higher risk for SUDEP, which may in turn inform strategies to reduce epilepsy-related deaths.

Gene therapy

Seizures do not respond to medication in as many as one-third of people with epilepsy, and unwanted side effects may occur in those whose treatment successfully controls seizures. Promising breakthroughs in gene therapy may provide hope for many people living with epilepsy. Researchers are designing types of gene therapy that are 'activated' when seizures occur.[18] To do this, they are investigating exactly which types of brain cell are active during seizures and how the molecules inside these cells change in people with epilepsy. Based on this new knowledge, a gene therapy could be designed to target these molecules during seizures. The rest of the time, when seizures do not occur, the gene therapy would be switched off and do nothing to the brain. This new technique could hugely refine the treatment of drug-resistant epilepsies. Excitingly, it could represent a 'one-off' treatment, so that people with epilepsy no longer require frequent and/or multiple medications to control their seizures.

Epilepsy and climate change

In 2020, epilepsy researchers, clinicians and climate-change scientists from around the world came together to form the Epilepsy and Climate Change (EpiCC) group. EpiCC has systematically analyzed the impact of climate change on people with epilepsy and the effects of epilepsy on climate change.[19]. For example, it is well known that temperature changes, particularly excessive heat, can be a potent trigger for seizures in DS. Anecdotally, many more people with epilepsy may be similarly affected. Conversely, patients travelling to clinics and professionals travelling to conferences contribute to global carbon emissions.

The global coronavirus (COVID-19) pandemic has demonstrated that it is possible to provide people with epilepsy with remote clinical care; indeed, in some cases it is desirable. A preliminary study in the UK has suggested that as many as 70% of people with epilepsy may prefer remote consultations in the long term.[20] Telemedicine could also provide expert healthcare to people in the developing world who may not be able to attend clinics hundreds of miles from where they live. Similarly, online education has developed markedly over the past few years. EpiCC ran the first global conference on epilepsy and climate change remotely in 2021.

Key points – research directions

- AI in the form of computer algorithms and wearable devices is being utilized to improve epilepsy diagnosis and care.
- PPI in epilepsy research is giving people with epilepsy a greater say in what research is undertaken, ensuring that funding goes into the research that matters most to them.
- In Canada, a national survey of people with epilepsy identified the top three research priorities to be the use of genetic markers in diagnosis and treatment, the long-term effects of ASM and the long-term impacts of seizures on the brain, overall health and development.
- Sophisticated network analysis is being applied to international MRI and EEG data to try to better understand the cause of SUDEP.
- Gene therapy, which is activated when seizures occur and switches off the rest of the time, has the potential to provide a one-off treatment for people with epilepsy, avoiding the need for frequent and/or multiple medications.
- The success of remote consultations for people with epilepsy and virtual conferences for epilepsy health professionals in recent years is likely to mean they will continue to be utilized in future.

References

1. The EPSET Project. www.epsetproject.org, last accessed 21 March 2022.
2. Bender E. Accelerating the diagnosis of epilepsy with computer modelling. Nature, 2021.www.nature.com/articles/d41586-021-01666-9, last accessed 21 March 2022.
3. Hashemi M, Vattikonda AN, Sip V et al. The Bayesian virtual epileptic patient: a probabilistic framework designed to infer the spatial map epileptogenicity in a personalized large-scale brain model of epilepsy spread. *Neuroimage* 2020;217:116839.

4. Epihunter. Invisible seizures now visible. www.epihunter.com, last accessed 21 March 2022.

5. Böttcher S, Bruno E, Manyakov NV et al. Detecting tonic-clonic seizures in multimodal biosignal data from wearables: methodology design and validation. *JMIR Mhealth Uhealth* 2021;9:e27674.

6. UNEEG Medical. Epilepsy: reliable seizure tracking. www.uneeg.com, last accessed 21 March 2022.

7. Byteflies. EpiCare@Home, 2022. www.byteflies.com/epicarehome, last accessed 21 March 2022.

8. Neuroevent Labs: Nelli. By experts, for experts. www.neuroeventlabs.com/for-physicians, last accessed 21 March 2022.

9. MES-CoBraD. The MES-CoBraD solution. www.mes-cobrad.eu/the-MES-CoBraD-solution, last accessed 21 March 2022.

10. Hughes M, Duffy C. Public involvement in health and social sciences research: a concept analysis. *Health Expect* 2018; 21:1183–90.

11. Reynolds J, Beresford R. "An active, productive life": narratives of, and through, participation in public and patient involvement in health research. *Qual Health Res* 2020;30:2265–77.

12. Singh A, Woelfle R, Chepesiuk R et al. Canadian epilepsy priority-setting partnership: toward a new national research agenda. *Epilepsy Behav* 2022;130:108673.

13. Epilepsy Research UK. *UK Epilepsy Priority Setting Partnership (PSP)*. www.epilepsyresearch.org.uk/uk-epilepsy-psp, last accessed 21 March 2022.

14. Epilepsy Research UK. Have Your Say – Shape Epilepsy Research Network. www.epilepsyresearch.org.uk/alifeinterrupted/shape-network,, last accessed 21 March 2022.

15. Epilepsy Research UK. Big Data – Bringing Information and People Together. www.epilepsyresearch.org.uk/our-research/research-blog/epilepsy-and-big-data, last accessed 18 March 2022.

16. Epilepsy Research UK. Assessing When and Why Epilepsy Treatment Fails to Work. www.epilepsyresearch.org.uk/research_portfolio/assessing-when-and-why-epilepsy-treatment-fails-to-work, last accessed 18 March 2022.

17. Epilepsy Research UK. Identifying the markers of SUDEP using global patient data. www.epilepsyresearch.org.uk/research_portfolio/identifying-the-markers-of-sudep-using-global-patient-data, accessed 18 March 2022.

18. Epilepsy Research UK. Using microRNA biosignatures as sensors for precision gene therapy. www.epilepsyresearch.org.uk/research_portfolio/using-biosignature-sensors-for-gene-therapy, last accessed 18 March 2022.

19. Gulcebi MI, Bartolini E, Lee O et al. Climate change and epilepsy: insights from clinical and basic science studies. *Epilepsy Behav* 2021;116:107791.

20. Bose S, Tittensor S, Greenhill L et al. Do patients' pre-pandemic clinic experiences influence their preference for remote consultations? Poster presentation, International League Against Epilepsy British Branch Scientific Virtual Meeting 2021.

Useful Resources

American Academy of Neurology
www.aan.com

American Epilepsy Society
www.aesnet.org

Association of British Neurologists
www.theabn.org

Brainwave
www.brainwave.org.uk

International Bureau for Epilepsy
www.ibe-epilepsy.org

International League Against Epilepsy
www.ilae.org

Canadian Epilepsy Alliance
www.canadianepilepsyalliance.org

Epilepsy Action (UK)
www.epilepsy.org.uk

Epilepsy Foundation (USA)
www.epilepsy.com

Epilepsy Scotland
www.epilepsyscotland.org.uk

Epilepsy Society (UK)
www.epilepsysociety.org.uk

Epilepsy Nurses Association (ESNA)
www.esna-online.org

FND Guide
www.neurosymptoms.org

Joint Epilepsy Council (UK)
www.jointepilepsycouncil.org.uk

Non-Epileptic Attacks
www.nonepilepticattacks.info

SUDEP Action (UK)
www.sudep.org

International guidelines
www.aan.com/professionals/practice/guideline

www.ilae.org/Vistors/Centre/Guidelines.cfm

www.nice.org.uk/guidance/ng217

https://www.sign.ac.uk/our-guidelines/

Driving regulations
Australia and New Zealand
www.austroads.com.au/publications/assessing-fitness-to-drive/ap-g56/neurological-conditions/seizures-and-epilepsy

www.epilepsy.org.au/about-epilepsy/living-with-epilepsy/lifestyle-issues/driving

Canada
www.canadianepilepsyalliance.org/about-epilepsy/living-with-epilepsy/driving

Europe
www.ibe-epilepsy.org/driving-regulations-task-force-2/

UK
www.epilepsysociety.org.uk/living-epilepsy/driving-and-epilepsy

www.gov.uk/epilepsy-and-driving

USA
www.epilepsy.com/lifestyle/driving-and-transportation/laws

Appendix 1: Treatment algorithm for tonic–clonic SE in adults in hospital

Initial patient management (0–5 minutes)

- Protect the patient; do not restrain
- Consider airway adjunct
- Administer oxygen
- Place patient in semiprone position, head down
- Gain i.v. access
- Obtain blood glucose.
- **If hypoglycemic**

Give 150–200mL 10% glucose i.v. stat

If seizures continue repeat this step and start 10% glucose infusion at 100mL/h

If suspicion of excess alcohol or malnutrition, give parenteral vitamin supplementation i.v before glucose replacement

First-line treatment (5–15 minutes)

If i.v. access	If no i.v. access
Dose 1: i.v. lorazepam 4mg bolus	**Dose 1: buccal midazolam 10mg** (alternative: midazolam 10mg i.m.)
Wait 5 minutes	Wait 5 minutes
Dose 2: i.v. lorazepam 4mg bolus	**Dose 2: buccal midazolam 10mg** (alternative: midazolam 10mg i.m.)
Wait 5 minutes	Wait 5 minutes

Use caution when prescribing multiple agents with similar mechanisms of action in view of potential adverse effects

Ongoing management
- Regular observations
- 12-lead ECG
- Obtain FBC, U&Es, LFTs, calcium, magnesium, clotting studies and, if applicable, ASM levels and blood gas
- Treat acidosis if severe (discuss with critical care)
- Determine if epilepsy has been diagnosed, medication history and acute seizure care plan
- Consider neuroimaging and EEG
- Consider possibility of PNES

Consider and treat potential causes
- Medication related (poor adherence, poor absorption, recent ASM changes, medication interactions or subtherapeutic levels)
- Infection
- Electrolyte disturbance
- Toxicity or drug withdrawal (including alcohol withdrawal)
- CNS pathology (e.g. tumor, stroke, encephalitis, PRES, neurodegenerative diseases)

If seizure not terminated after 15 minutes move to second-line treatment

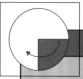

Second-line treatment (15 minutes onwards)

i.v. or i.o. access
Escalate to critical care* as per local policy

Dose 3:
  – **LEV, 60 mg/kg i.v., maximum 4500mg (over 10 minutes)**
OR
  – **PHT, 20mg/kg i.v., maximum 2g**
  (50mg/min, 25mg/min for elderly or patients with cardiac history)

> **Caution**: PHT administration requires cardiac monitoring and wide bore i.v. access, as risk of extravasation and phlebitis

OR
  – **VPA, 40mg/kg i.v., maximum 3000mg (over 5 minutes)**

	Preferred if	Avoid if
LEV	• Polypharmacy (fewest drug interactions)	• Mood or behavioral disorder (may worsen symptoms)
PHT		• Cardiac monitoring not available • Known or suspected generalized epilepsy (GGE) • Hypotension/bradycardia/heart block • Porphyria • Known or suspected overdose of recreational drugs/alcohol withdrawal
VPA	• Known or suspected idiopathic generalized epilepsy (GGE) • Comorbid mood disorder/migraines	• **Women of childbearing potential (consider pregnancy test)** • Liver disease • Pancreatitis • Known or suspected metabolic disorder/ mitochondrial disease (risk of hepatotoxicity)

Dose 4:
If seizure has not stopped after completion of infusion consider second i.v. infusio of a different ASM from the same list (LEV, PHT, VPA) or PB.

PB can be given at 15mg/kg as a single dose, maximum rate 100mg/min.

If seizure is terminated:
• ABCDE assessment of patient at regular intervals
• Escalate to critical care setting if indicated*
• Start supportive medical care and look for underlying cause of SE

If seizure not terminated at any point > 30minutes since seizure onset move to third-line treatment

Third-line treatment (30 minutes onwards)

The following stages must have anesthetic input, airway support and early arrangements for transfer to critical care unit*

General anesthesia – induction and maintenance

Consider the properties of each drug when selecting induction and maintenance agents (these may be different)

	Induction	Maintenance
Propofol	1–2mg/kg bolus	Up to 4mg/kg/h titrated to effect; continuous infusion for minimum 24 hours
Thiopental sodium	3–5mg/kg bolus	3–5mg/kg/h titrated to effect; continuous infusion for minimum 24hours
Ketamine	3mg/kg bolus	1mg/kg/h titrated to effect,maximum 10mg/kg/h; continuous infusion for minimum 24 hours
Midazolam	0.2mg/kg bolus	0.05–0.5mg/kg/h titrated to effect; continuous infusion for minimum 24 hours

- General anesthesia maintenance is typically with propofol and/or midazolam in the first instance
- If first maintenance agent is unsuccessful at terminating seizures, use second anesthetic agent
- As a minimum, perform intermittent EEG, aiming for suppression of electrographic epileptic activity
- Maintenance doses of ASM (start 10–14 hours after loading dose to allow regular ongoing dosing)

Caution

- Be aware that **midazolam** exhibits multiple drug interactions
- Monitor patients on **propofol** for propofol infusion syndrome (metabolic acidosis, rhabdomyolysis, renal failure, hypertriglyceridemia, refractory bradycardia and cardiac failure)
- Be aware that interpretation of processed EEG monitoring,such as bispectral index, may become unreliable when using **ketamine** infusion

Fourth-line treatment (24+ hours)

Treatment at this stage should be guided by specialists using an MDT approach. There is no high-quality RCT evidence to guide treatment decisions.

- Look for an **underlying cause and treat** (e.g. infectious/autoimmune encephalitis, systemic infection, electrolyte disturbance, toxicity)
- **Neurosurgical intervention** (e.g. lesional resection)
- If no underlying cause identified in first presentation of seizures, consider **immunotherapy**: high-dose steroids, IVIG and/or therapeutic plasmapheresis
- **Alternative treatments** include therapeutic hypothermia, ketogenic diet and magnesium infusion
- **Discontinue ineffective treatments** to minimize risk of adverse effects

*Management in critical care unit
- Give all patients an up-to-date ECG on admission to critical care
- Ensure continued treatment with regular ASM, prescribed alongside any additional treatment as part of this pathway
- Document why treatment decisions have been made and ensure detailed communication with next of kin regarding treatment plan and prognosis

---

ABCDE, airway, breathing, circulation, disability, exposure; FBC, full blood count; i.m., intramuscular; i.o., intraosseus; i.v., intravenous; IVIG, intravenous immunoglobulin; LFT, liver function test; MDT, multidisciplinary team; PRES, posterior reversible encephalopathy syndrome; RCT, randomized controlled trial; U&E, urea and electrolytes.

Reproduced with permission from Mitchell J, Adan G, Whitehead C, Musial G, Bennett R, Burness C. *Status Epilepticus Guideline*, version 1.1. The Walton Centre NHS Foundation Trust, 2020. www.thewaltoncentre.nhs.uk/pathways.htm

INDEX